When The Music Stopped I Kept On Dancing

Also by Angela Riggs

Voices of the Prairie

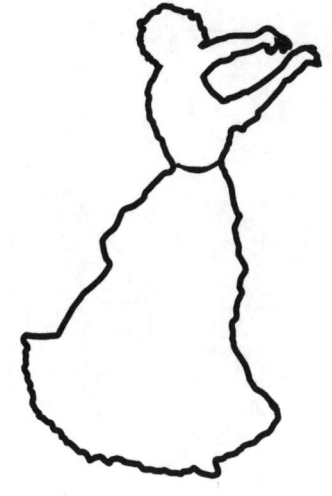

*This book is my gift to everyone
who has to learn to live with limitations.*

Angela Riggs

When The Music Stopped I Kept On Dancing

A Story of Courage, Hope and the Magnificence of the Human Spirit

Angela Riggs

BookPartners, Inc.
Wilsonville, Oregon

Copyright 1995 by Angela Riggs
All rights reserved
Printed in U.S.A.
Library of Congress Catalog 94-78434
ISBN 1-885221-19-3

This book may not be reproduced in whole or in part, by mimeograph or any other means, without permission. For information contact:

BookPartners, Inc.
P. O. Box 922
Wilsonville, Oregon 97070

Dedication

*To Wayne,
my lifelong dancing partner.*

Acknowledgements

Encouragement for writing this book came from many sources. Jim Kapron planted the seed in my mind and gently nudged it along to make it grow. Theresa Ripley was my sounding board and a tireless cheer leader. Caye, Pat, Merry and dozens of other friends convinced me that my story might inspire others. I am grateful to my editor, Ursula Bacon, whose skill and humor made completing this book a pleasant experience. Thorn Bacon contributed his professional knowledge and gave me the necessary assurances for this project.

Appreciation goes to Evelyn Frank who added substance to her constant encouragement by proofreading the final manuscript. I will always be grateful to Bill and Betty O'Hearn who gave new meaning to the word "caring."

Special thanks to my husband, my children and grandchildren who stood staunchly by me and made me believe I can do anything I set out to do.

Angela Riggs

Table of Contents

Prologue .1
Chapter One 9
Chapter Two 21
Chapter Three 29
Chapter Four 45
Chapter Five 55
Chapter Six 69
Chapter Seven 75
Chapter Eight 85
Chapter Nine 99
Chapter Ten 107
Chapter Eleven 121
Chapter Twelve 135
Chapter Thirteen 155
Chapter Fourteen 161
Epilogue 167

Do not go gentle into that good night,
Old age should burn and rave at close of day;
Rage, rage against the dying of the light.
— *Dylan Thomas*

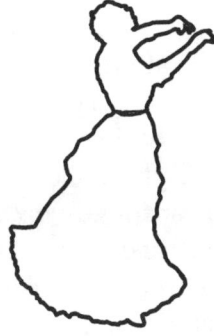

Prologue

> Life is what happens to you
> when you're making other plans.
> *Betty Talmadge*

I have amyotrophic lateral sclerosis — ALS for short. You probably don't know what that is.

I didn't either, until those dreadful three words of medical terminology became my label, my sentence — my personal scarlet letter.

Amyotrophic lateral sclerosis is more commonly known as ALS or Lou Gehrig's disease. It is a neuromuscular disease which causes gradual degeneration of the voluntary muscles and ultimately leaves the victim completely helpless. It becomes fatal when the respiratory and swallowing muscles no longer function. The disease does not affect the brain, the eyes, or hearing and the average life span for ALS victims is two to five years after diagnosis.

Cause unknown.

Cure unknown.

As I am writing this story, this insidious and disabling

disease has taken control of my life: I am unable to pick up a book, raise a fork to my mouth, take a brisk walk in the fresh air — or for that matter, walk even one step in my living room — reach for a tissue which is within an inch of my grasp, help myself to a hot buttered roll from the basket in the middle of the dining room table. I cannot give my grandchildren a hug or dance with my husband to our favorite tunes of the forties. I can't bake a batch of my special Ranger oatmeal-raisin cookies. I cannot turn over in my bed, or cook up a simple meal of stew and cornbread.

Every day is fraught with frustration.

I am no longer independent. Independence is but a memory of another time, another world. I just know one thing: I must keep on, I will not give up.

Even though I mourn for what I've lost, I never stop reminding myself of what I've gained from having experienced those losses. I had taken my life for granted. Good health, our comfortable, active and pleasant retirement lifestyle, I had considered my due. All that changed when I was diagnosed with ALS ten years ago.

I have learned to treasure the simplest things — a friend taking me for a Sunday drive in the country to see the brilliant autumn colors; a shopping trip to the mall where the sign "Classy Chassis" on the back of my power wheelchair brings a smile to harried, hurrying shoppers; sharing a lasagna dinner with our daughter Judy and grandchildren, John and Susan.

I treasure a visit on the telephone with our son, Larry, his wife, Lori and our grandchildren, Kristine and Brad who live in far-away Wisconsin. These calls provide me with strength and closeness that even 2,000 miles of separation cannot dilute or divide.

Attempting to compare the gains to the losses in my

life would be like comparing apples to oranges — each ranks tops in its own category. Would I have ever made time to write two books if I had not been forced to curtail my physical activities? Would I have freely exchanged my golf clubs for a computer? Would I have turned the housekeeping chores over to help, (caring and competent as they are), as well as to my husband who had to awaken his cooking and caregiving talents that had lain dormant somewhere in the recesses of his male persona?

As I count the gains, it would seem they far outweigh the losses, I think. Or is my glowing appraisal of these losses merely an accommodating act to ease my despair for having had to trade what I no longer can do for some new experiences which I have come to view as even more satisfying and unique? Perhaps so. The mind does strange and wonderful things.

After the initial shock and the accompanying depression of my ALS diagnosis began to ebb, I knew I had to get started on the rest of my life. The two-to-five-year life/death sentence which went with the diagnosis of ALS would bring the kind of life I had known to an abrupt halt. I would not have a lot of time to do what was important to me. The prognosis became the propelling force to begin writing before the muscles in my body completely deteriorated.

Writing about my husband's and my childhood on the farm in Nebraska was something I had always wanted to do but somehow just never got around to doing. If ever there was a right time, it was right then — right now.

I buckled down, began at the beginning, pecked away at it, and gave life to a family history titled, *Memories into Memoirs* which became a legacy — something of value. It was my gift to our four grandchildren and the next generations, as well as for our twenty nieces and nephews who all grew up close to our farm homes. They all received a hardbound book of the family story highlighted by reproductions of old family photos. In years to come, they can relive their own "good old days" and engage in lively "I remember when" reminiscing.

In spite of the dark cloud hovering over my head, time flew by and before I knew it, there was a pleasant and encouraging surprise in store for me.

My five-year life-death sentence was up and there I was, still mobile and on most days still brimming over with a boundless zest for living. There was so much left for me to do before my muscles turned to an inert mass of inactivity — to a blob of nothing. The gruesome statistics were the irrefutable proof of what lay in store for the victims of the disease. Sadly, I had seen it in the ALS patients we encountered in our group support meetings which Wayne and I attended.

Slowly, ever so slowly but surely, changes were taking place in my body. I was preparing for the inevitable. I had regressed from walking with one cane to using two. Before long my wobbly legs demanded yet more support and a walker became a necessity. It did make me feel more secure but I wasn't thrilled about the extra appendage. No one had to draw me a picture to know what lay ahead.

The walker served me well for around the house; however, being a social animal, I needed to be independent enough to roam around the neighborhood. I liked to visit friends, or just get out of the house to see a sunset, admire the azaleas and rhododendrons which celebrated yet another glorious spring in the Willamette Valley of Oregon. Since I could no longer drive an automobile, a three-wheel scooter was the partial answer to maintaining some form of independence.

I became the owner and operator of a motorized chair, dubbed "Classy Chassis." Friends jazzed up my wheels with hand-painted flowers, pieces of lace around the basket, ribbons on the handlebars, and in direct contrast with the friendly frou-frou, my motorcycle friend, Skip, added a bumper sticker that boasted boldly, "I'd rather be riding my Harley." I had regained a piece of my independence.

Five years later, as muscles deteriorated further, it became necessary to look for another type of conveyance to make life as "normal" as possible for me. A power wheelchair was the answer, and after a decade of having ALS, the distant cousin of my Classy Chassis became my new, highly-valued and reliable companion — complete with signs and stickers.

I was fortunate that my right hand and arm had not forsaken me entirely. I was still able to type, in a manner of speaking, (using one finger and/or thumb and still later, supporting my right arm with my left, grasping a pencil — eraser-side down) to hit the keys of my computer keyboard, one letter at a time.

Hey, it was better than nothing!

Confucius say: "Consider the turtle, he moves forward only when he sticks his neck out." Was I ever sticking my neck out!

So what next? I feel like I've been granted a stay of execution. An entire decade had gone by and here I am, still rattling around. Living with ALS isn't easy, but sometimes when I look around me, I think that just being alive is a special kind of bravery.

I decided to use the borrowed time to start another writing project and a story that had been scurrying around in my head. For years I've had an interest in genealogy and spent many hours in the libraries in various cities, tracing my ancestry. I owned a green file case bulging with hard-to-find data and all sorts of information about my family. It seemed a shame not to put that material in story form for future generations to have.

The idea for a book broiled up in my mind with the force of a pressure cooker about to blow its lid. That's what I had to do — write a book in novel style based on the reams of factual information stowed away in my green file. At age 70, I began one of the most exciting and satisfying times of my life, in spite of the battle with the constantly weakening of my muscles.

I had all sorts of doubts and the project seemed to take on overwhelming proportions. But I knew there was just one way to get where I wanted to go.

I had to get started.

After four years of writing and rewriting — accomplished on my computer keyboard, with a pencil clutched in my fingers, the left hand supporting the right tapping out letters to make words, I finished my book, *Voices of the Prairie*. My modest print run of 1,600 copies is now in the hands of readers all over the United States, as well as in Germany, New Zealand and Canada.

I could hardly believe that the writing, followed by the successful marketing of my book, would ever be a part of my ALS-affected life. I really felt I had accomplished something. I was thrilled.

I remembered the words of Eleanor Roosevelt who so modestly stated, "... as for accomplishments, I just did what I had to do as things came along."

For some unknown reason, I had started to keep a journal in 1981, two years before ALS symptoms began to appear. I had no inkling my brief journal entries would become the basis for this present book which I began in

1993 — not just as a tiresome accounting of living with a crippling killer disease, but as a testimony to the undefeatable qualities of the human spirit I share with the rest of humanity, and the fact that all things in life are possible. That goes for me and holds true for you.

I want this book to speak to everyone who has to face seemingly insurmountable adversities in whatever form or shape they come. I want people to understand that it is life that counts. How we deal with serious problems, how we handle disappointments and heartbreaks, and how fully we live each day is what brings the color to the sunset, unquenchable joy to meet the next sunrise, and robs death of its tragedy.

When The Music Stopped, I Kept On Dancing is dedicated to all whose problems at times seem unbearable. At the risk of repeating myself, I want my message to be strong and clear:

It is the manner in which we cope with circumstances that makes the difference, not only within ourselves but to those around us.

I want people to understand that we CAN stretch beyond our arm's length, reach beyond the limiting horizons of our afflictions and live up to our limitless potential. We all have what it takes to wrestle with the dragons in our lives.

The diseases that burden our existence and inflict their hideously crippling and maiming effects on our bodies may not be fair, but the ability to make the best of every moment — to make that jug of lemonade out of the lemons of life — that gift we all have. It's up to us to use it.

And when we remove ourselves from our personal tragedies and crises and make room to help others, we reinforce and validate our existence regardless of our physical condition.

We may no longer be able to do things for ourselves, but we all have the power to give joy to those whose lives we touch — no matter how briefly. Our actions and our feelings have the facility to reach out like ripples upon the water, spreading pleasure and love all around — and, we as the center of giving, derive the greatest benefits. The gift of joy comes back twofold.

So, remember, when the music stops, keep on dancing to the melody in your heart.

Angela Riggs

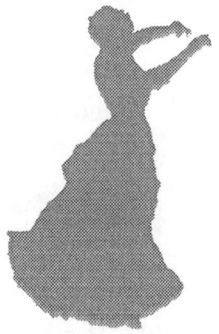

Chapter One

We all live in suspense from day to day from hour to hour;
In other words, we are the hero of our own story.
Mary McCarthy

In spite of the fact that the summer of 1983 was a bit cool and late in coming, the greens were lush and thick, and the flowers around the houses, edging the walks and gracing the neighbors' gardens, were bright and in full bloom. On that day in July we had typical Oregon weather — the sun darted in and out from behind low-sailing clouds and lingered just long enough to keep the temperature in the 70s. The air was mild and the afternoon breeze carried the fragrant scent of blossoms on its breath. It had been a perfect day for golf — and I had made good use of it.

I had played 18 holes with friends from the women's golf league and had fully enjoyed the game, the company and the day. Back at the house, after a quick shower and change, I poured myself a tall glass of iced tea and plopped down in a comfortable chair in our spacious living room whose big sliding glass door and windows looked out on the immaculate greens of the eighth hole of the Charbonneau golf course. There was lots of time before my husband, Wayne, would return from playing his round of golf that most probably would culminate in a leisurely stop at the club house — lots of time before thinking about preparing dinner.

The big door to the patio was halfway open and the sun-warmed, rose-scented afternoon air drifted gently around me. Life, indeed was wonderful. How lucky for Wayne and I to have found this beautiful spot, this friendly community, this "Garden of Eden," to enjoy our retirement years. And enjoy, we did. Wayne, of all people, deserved a time of leisure. He had done more than his share of hard work and nose-to-the-grindstone years, as well as serving his country in two wars.

At peace and at ease, I leaned back against the soft chair. Languidly I stretched my body, and felt my muscles respond — tighten and relax. A morning of walking and swinging a club at that little white ball was certainly a great exercise. I felt wonderful in the stillness of that summer day.

I watched a fat robin, with his skinny legs braced against the ground, pull an unlucky worm from its dark hiding place in the earth. A busy bee buzzed by and settled on a blossom as I let my thoughts wander the back roads of my memories — as far back as growing up on a Nebraska farm, where life had been simple, often sparse and not always easy. Now, surrounded by so many delightful friends and neighbors, I remembered the loneliness of living on a farm far from town, where a visit from the Watkins Man selling his genuine vanilla extract, spices and "stuff" would easily be the highlight of the month.

I left that lonely farm soon after I graduated from high school and ventured into the "big world," in Lincoln, the state capital. After attending business school for two years, I landed a job as a secretary. I liked my work and had made quite a few friends when I met tall and handsome Wayne Riggs on a blind date. He was a young teacher and coach at a school in a small town not far from Lincoln. I liked him immediately, and we started to date.

We soon discovered that we both loved to dance and rarely did we miss the opportunity to spend an evening dancing to the music of our times. Sometimes we termed our dance steps the *Nebraska Hop*, but, call it what you will, that man had rhythm — although he did jump a little high at times.

We went to all the big ballrooms scattered about Nebraska — some were out in the country, surrounded by a sea of corn fields smack in the middle of nowhere. Others were in the small towns where weddings were celebrated by hiring a band. It was customary for the bride in her white satin gown, and the groom in his new dark blue suit to lead the first dance, and it wasn't long before everyone moved and swayed in one fashion or another to the rhythm of the music.

In every ballroom, there was a huge, slowly rotating, mirrored ball suspended from the ceiling, casting about a thousand glittering, flitting rainbow lights which reflected on the dancers beneath its sparkling magic. It was the era of the big bands — sweet rhythm and sounds, and wonderful lyrics. Bands traveled from town to town, city to city and the dance halls were packed with couples gliding and twirling and bopping to the popular tunes. Before he became famous, Lawrence Welk brought his music to our small town, and the people who danced to his music that night won't ever forget it.

We were so young, and we had a wonderful time. We

didn't know any better!

It was pleasant looking out at the peaceful setting of green grass and tall pines as I continued my dreamy reverie and recalled our wedding some 40 years ago.

World War II was raging in Europe and Wayne joined the navy thinking he would complete his two-year stint and then return to civilian life, which, incidentally, included me. He was to leave within the month.

My cousin with whom I was living at the time, prepared a lovely farewell dinner for Wayne on a wintry Sunday in December in Lincoln, Nebraska. As the family gathered around the table someone had turned on the radio to a broadcast of Sammy Kaye and his band. In the middle of one of our favorite tunes there came a harsh interruption. The excited announcer's voice was laced with the importance of the message:

"The Japanese have bombed Pearl Harbor."

In stunned silence we looked at each other. War was now a different reality. War had come home. Our eyes turned to the centerpiece of our festive dinner table which held a small American flag — all lost for a moment in our own thoughts.

Two days later Wayne was gone. He had been called to report immediately to the Naval Training base in Norfolk, Virginia. After basic training he was transferred to Rhode Island. Our letters flew back and forth across the country and one day, an engagement ring arrived in the mail, followed by a phone call in which we set the date for our wedding. I hung up the phone and let go with a resounding yell of excitement.

I was going to marry the man I loved.

I grabbed a map to look up just where Newport, Rhode Island was. My finger came to rest on a tiny spot on the map no bigger than my thumb nail — tucked away close to the northeast shore of the Atlantic Ocean.

Wherever it was, I was going. And, I was going alone.

Mother gave a bridal shower for me, I packed a trunk with my few earthly possessions which included a carefully folded, simple, white wedding dress and told my family goodbye. I double-checked my detailed train schedule and was off to discover an unknown world and a new life. I rode the swaying, bumpy train halfway across America with never a doubt in my mind I was doing the right thing.

The interminable train ride finally ended and when I stepped down to the platform, I looked about and saw Wayne's lanky frame towering over the crowd. He looked taller and so handsome in his navy uniform. I remember my blue hat flying off my head as I ran into his open arms.

People in uniforms and in civilian garb thronged about us, some were greeting loved ones with big hugs, while others said their tearful goodbyes embracing each other to the last moment. In spite of the seriousness of war, and all of life's uncertainties, there was a kind of romance, a kind of excitement about it all.

Without elaborate wedding plans, Wayne and I were married on June 13, 1942 in the Navy Chapel on the base in a simple ceremony.

For two years he was stationed at different naval bases. We were quick to move and I followed him to Bloomington, Indiana, to Gulfport, Mississippi and New Orleans, cherishing every moment we were able to spend together. Sooner or later, he would be shipped out to sea.

When his orders finally came, there was nothing else for me to do but return to Nebraska. I would get a job and like thousands of other women in times of war face a period of loneliness and worry, never knowing where he was and how he was, and if he'd come back in one piece.

I learned that his ship would return to the east coast about every six weeks. As soon as his ship was in he called, and I managed to get a train reservation. I had made a friend out of the Burlington man, and twice I made the long trek to meet my husband. I still remember how excited I was to be in big New York City — me, a farm girl from Nebraska.

I brought my self back into the present for a brief moment, looked around our lovely home that summer afternoon, refilled my glass of iced tea and remembered those early struggles after the war — a dingy apartment, little money, our first baby, no refrigerator, no washing machine — no nothing. Times were tough, trying to adjust from military to civilian life. But Wayne had a job, and I was grateful for having him back alive and unharmed.

But I do remember our humble beginnings:

Wayne was a college basketball coach in a small town in Nebraska. There just was no place to rent, and the three of us (by then we had a baby son) moved into the basement of the college infirmary. I worked on making the cement block walls of our basement look homey. But even the brightly printed flour-sack curtains did nothing to relieve the stark grey of the walls, mainly because I knew no way to attach them to the unyielding cement.

The baby crib filled the "bedroom" (formerly a storage closet) and crab-like, we had to walk sideways to gain access to the cubicle. Our refrigerator was a tin box placed outside the front door — it just wasn't Better Homes & Gardens. In spite of it all, our little family of three was warm and secure with a roof overhead and the war was over.

Wayne decided on a career change, ventured into the business world, and we moved to Iowa City, Iowa. We bought an old house and made an adventure out of refurbishing it. Our daughter was born in that old house and completed our happy family circle.

I loved working around our home and being with the children. I took care of them, played their games — I was still a kid myself. Having been raised on a farm had instilled in me a sense of equanimity. I had learned to take things in stride, to "make do" with what life had to offer and to enjoy the simple things. In the ensuing years, we made several moves and each one not only brought us to a different part of the country but presented new opportunities for Wayne, who, in the meantime had finished his doctorate.

With one interruption — the Korean War — he stayed in the field of education and advanced from teacher to principal, and finally became a superintendent. He spent the last 23 years of his career as superintendent of schools in Nebraska and Illinois.

The years seemed to have passed with the same swiftness as the fading of a lovely day. The afternoon shadows lengthened in readiness for evening to fall. I recalled Wayne's decision to retire early, and how at the same time I left my 10-year career of selling real estate. Wayne had worked very hard for so many years. But times had changed the school systems drastically, and he felt it was the perfect moment to move on to the next stage in life. He retired.

A trip to Oregon to visit our daughter brought us to Charbonneau. We saw, we fell in love — Oregon conquered our hearts, and we bought our home all in the same day.

We returned to Illinois, put our house on the market, and worried a little if we had done the right thing. We had made a spur-of-the-moment decision that just might backfire on us. But of course, we had done the right thing. We felt so fortunate to have stumbled onto this delightful community near Portland with its beautifully groomed grounds and facilities and, above all, we delighted in those wonderful people who became part of our lives.

Wayne and I took advantage of our newly-found freedom, and managed to fill our daily agenda with all sorts of activities. We squeezed in as much golf as possible, and spent a lot of time enjoying the outdoors.

We explored the beautiful Oregon coast, walked the beaches for miles, and strolled through the small coastal towns that hovered at the edges of the sandy shores of the Pacific Ocean. Everyone was friendly and hospitable.

We visited our daughter, Judy, who lived a short hour's drive away. It was a joy to have John and Susan, our small grandchildren, all to ourselves while their parents took time off. The children added spark and pleasure to our lives. After watching their antics and enjoying their endearing yet so different personalities to the fullest, we would exercise the time-honored grandparents' right and send them home a bit spoiled and happy, hoping they would keep a few fond memories of the time spent with us.

We took time to travel, and renewed World War II friendships that were forty years old. Living on the West Coast ourselves, we didn't have that far to go. We visited long-time friends in Monterey, California and in Clarkston, Washington, where our host's home in the canyon overlooked the Snake River at its confluence with the Clearwater River.

There we stood at the spot where the Lewis and Clark expedition was said to have had a feast with the Indian tribes of centuries ago. We walked the ruts of the Oregon Trail ten years before the commemoration of the 150th anniversary of the emigrants' trek to the lush Willamette Valley. Thanks to the pioneers breaking the trail, we now lived in this wonderful land with all its bountiful gifts. No matter what afflictions and challenges come our way, how fleeting our existence on this earth may be — the land will always be there in all its splendor. And as long as we breathe, we have the privilege and opportunity to enjoy its beauty and be comforted by its timelessness.

One of my dreams came true in 1980 when I decided to go to Europe. I was going to visit Austria and Germany, including the village of Haaren, where my ancestors lived in the early 1800s. This was where my years of research came to life. I visited the very spot where my ancestors were born and raised more than a century ago. My family's 1655 stone and timber home was still in excellent condition. Its thick walls and sturdy beams had well withstood the elements, the people and the times. It was from that old house in Haaren that my grandfather and his brother left for America and began their perilous journey to their new home.

They settled in the untamed prairie of the Nebraska Territory along with other pioneers. Today, the old farmstead in Nebraska is still in the family. I thought that my crossing the Atlantic and setting foot on German soil at the birthplace of my ancestors was completing the circle. After three weeks of touring the countryside, gawking at glorious cathedrals, attending an authentic Octoberfest and watching the famous Oberammergau Passion play — which is put on only once every ten years by the people of Oberammergau — I returned home full of ideas for my genealogy book.

It took no time for me to settle back into our comfortable routine, and between visits with our neighbors and friends, playing bridge, golf, gardening and enjoying the outdoors, the days just flew by. Wayne and I went for long walks, attended dances at the club, or stayed put with a good book. We loved our home, celebrated life and counted our blessings.

I agreed with whoever coined the phrase: "God is at the wheel of the Universe, and all's well with the world."

All was certainly well in my world.

Well, almost all.

Some seemingly inconsequential thing rankled and perplexed me. It bothered me enough, that I confided my concern to my journal several days later. I made the following brief entry:

July, 1983
Left forefinger muscle gone. Does not respond when I try to point finger or move it upward.

Like most women who have taken care of a family all their lives, nursed sick kids night and day, helped with the neighbors when they themselves need looking after, they ignore the little things. I paid little attention to my finger, something I considered a minor health nuisance. Everything comes to pass, nothing comes to stay. I knew that nobody ever died of a cold in the nose, and discomforts went away with the scrubbing of the kitchen floor. Anything that didn't shriek with pain seemed to disappear when one's attention was directed at something more important. Nothing heroic about that. It's just the way mothers are!

I had never been one to spend much time on self examination, for probing the recesses of my soul, but I realized that I was a bit uneasy when I discovered my left index finger was not working the way it was supposed to. As a matter of fact it did nothing — it just flopped about.

I made an appointment with a hand specialist who came highly recommended. Doctor X looked at my hand, bent it slowly backwards and forwards, checked my finger, moved it here, moved there, let it drop, picked it up and did it all over again. After thinking about it for a second or two, he diagnosed my willy-nilly finger as having a ruptured tendon, which, in case there was no improvement, could be repaired with surgery. The whole examination including the brilliant diagnosis took less than three minutes, yet our bill — which we paid on our way out — came to $72.

I accepted this splendid and seemingly simple solution to my problem. I was relieved, went home, and sat back waiting for my "ruptured" tendon to regain its proper state of well-being.

I waited. Nothing happened. My finger remained unresponsive. When I played golf and my hands grasped the club, my forefinger would not curl and settle in its place, but kept flopping about. When engaged in any action that required all five fingers of my left hand to do their bidding, all but that finger obeyed. Still, I didn't pay much attention to it and continued to enjoy the summer days.

August, 1983
Left leg weak under stress, such as fast walking. Difficulty in raising from chair which I had already noticed a year ago.
What is happening to my muscles?

Wayne and I walked the grounds daily in the cool, early morning hours and sometimes we ventured out for a long walk on sun-drenched afternoons. At times I noticed that I had difficulty keeping up with my husband's easy stride which my body had always automatically matched inch for inch. I realized that I sometimes dragged my left foot, and that I had a slight problem picking it off of the ground. This would never do. I beefed up my exercise program. I walked up and down stairs to strengthen my leg muscles.

I wasn't overly concerned and chalked it up to being tired — or I was getting older. After all, nothing ever remains the same. Besides I was busy getting ready for a big trip. Another one of my dreams was about to come true.

I was going to China. I was so excited. Traveling the world was always on my mind. Sometimes I felt that I was straining at the bit to run and test and discover every inch of the globe. I have always had a curious mind. Maybe in my childhood, the endlessly waving fields of wheat and corn meeting the horizons of my world must have whispered to me what wonders lay beyond the limits of what my eyes could see.

Now I was going to visit another world on the other side of the globe. The same tour director with whom I had traveled to Europe casually mentioned to me that there was one place left with a group which would be touring China for three weeks. Would I like to go?

I said "Yes" so quickly I didn't realize I'd said it!

I was anxiously waiting for October to come around. I busied myself with the preparations for leaving the house in ship-shape condition, getting my traveling gear ready and catching up on some reading other than the travel brochures.

I forgot all about my silly finger and my reluctant left foot. I was on my way to adventure.

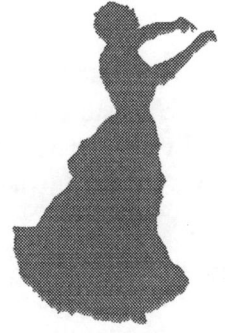

Chapter Two

> You can't be brave
> if you only had wonderful
> things happen to you.
> *Mary Tyler Moore*

We arrived in busy, noisy Shanghai — our first stop — on a bright, golden October day, and went by bus to Beijing. I marveled at the vastness of the land where the peasants tilled their fields in the same manner they had done for centuries. Hard, back-breaking work without the help of modern farm equipment had to produce a generous harvest to feed China's population of over one billion.

We looked and admired the traditional offering of goods from vendors clustered along the roadside. Things were done by hand, from delicate embroidery, to stone and ivory carvings, to ornamental filigree work.

The vast sky that stretched over the Great Wall which reached for miles and miles into the land, was a deep China-blue as far as the eye could see. The sun lay warm on the ancient landmark. Strange as the land was to me, I felt so much a part of it all.

The next day our tour guide took us to the Temple of Heaven, and as I walked down the many steps from this magnificent monument to deity, my left foot went out from under me, and I found myself sprawled out on the hard, unforgiving stone slabs.

My camera went flying in one direction and my dignity in the other. Instantly a dozen curious Chinese gathered about, and as I lay flat on my back, I looked up into a variety of concerned faces circling above me, hovering like sea gulls in preparation for a landing. Women and men of all ages, dressed in the uniform dark blue tunic of the day, chatted solicitations in their language foreign to me.

I tried to retrieve my camera, certain I could regain my dignity by sitting up on one of the rough steps. That's what I had intended. However, my first movement produced a sharp pain in my ankle, and as I looked down at my left foot, I was amazed to see that it had already swollen to almost double its normal size.

Li, our young and agile Chinese guide, literally flew to my rescue. Before I knew what was happening he nimbly hoisted me up, carried me piggyback down the steps, and when he reached the bottom, unceremoniously plunked me on the nearest bench. By that time I had no shred of dignity left, but it didn't matter. All I could think of was the pain, especially since Li was playing doctor, and rotated my ankle in order to determine if it was broken. If it had not been broken before, it undoubtedly would have been then.

It was October the 12th, 1983, when I sat on the hard cement bench, all alone, contemplating my fate. Our guide pushed the rest of the group of 23 eager American tourists ever onward to yet another Chinese wonder, the Hall of Echoes, led by the versatile Li, who demonstrated his agility by running backwards as fast as anyone in our group could run forward. When Li and the group came back to collect me, I was still staring glassy-eyed at my offending left foot, which seemed to be growing larger by the minute, and at this point resembled a purple balloon.

How could I have done such an absurd thing, I mourned to myself. Here I was on a once-in-a-lifetime trip taking a stupid fall on our third day out on this tour of China.

Well, at least I had walked the Great Wall the day before, so if I never saw another sight or walked another step I would still consider the trip a great success. I had purchased an ancient coin of heavy brass with a square hole in the middle, said to have been used a thousand years ago by the imperial dynasties. I bought a miniature cloisonne snuff pot and odd pieces of amber-colored jade. How could I have thought jade was always green?

My imagination ran rampant as I wondered about the people who might have had at one time owned these "rare finds." I was especially fascinated by the cloisonne snuff pot with its intricate design and graceful shape, its inside blackened by what surely must have been daily use by some great emperor of some mighty dynasty.

These thoughts ran through my head, along with shades of gloom and doom. How could I maneuver these hundreds of steps that seemed to be the trademark of this ancient land — 123 steps DOWN to the tomb of the Emperor of the Ming dynasty, followed by going UP those same 123 steps. That's when my left foot had started to feel weak and draggy, and that's when I met my downfall at the Temple of Heaven on that sunny, bright, 12th day of October 1983.

Nevertheless, the show must go on, and I spent the

remainder of my three-week tour of China and Japan hobbling on one foot with the support of crutches which I could not master, a decorative cane which our tour director found in the Friendship Store in Xian, and the strong arms of the men in our group. Indeed, two fellow travelers made a hand cradle and carried me up 73 steps to the train depot (why are train stations in China at the top of the very highest hill in the province?) where we rode the train to our next stop on this tour of wonders. We slept on hand-embroidered pillows filled with rice, and laughed hysterically while we women tried to conquer the eastern-style toilets, which consisted of nothing more than a hole in the floor.

Then there was the time when a wonderful Chinese man and woman put me on a baggage cart to transport me from one train station to the next, very carefully circumventing a post with a three-foot wide clearance which stood between the baggage cart and a drop-off of thirty feet. I looked down and thought my time had come. What was I doing here in China on a baggage cart being hauled like a sack of rice, staring down into the chasm of a thirty-foot drop?

Even as I watched the concerned faces of my Chinese drivers, I prayed the wheel would not catch the edge of the post and overturn the cart. I was destined to live and carry on. Finally we made it to the place where the rest of the tour group was waiting. They shouted a joyful "hallelujah," applauded my Chinese saviors, got out their cameras and amid flashbulbs popping shouted the cutline for their photographic efforts: "Angie on a baggage cart in China!" Clearly, it's the unexpected that adds zing to our lives.

Arriving at Xian, produced the first opportunity to have my foot X-rayed for a possible break. Xian is a popular tourist spot because it is the place where a terra cotta "army" of men were planted underground to protect their emperor in his grave at the top of the hill a thousand years ago.

English-speaking Chinese guides were hard to find on the day our tour group landed in Xian, and consequently we ended up with a guide who spoke no English. Here I was, being taken to the outskirts of goodness-knows-where with a guide who did not speak English, to a Chinese doctor whose expertise lay in performing acupuncture with his thumbs, until I yelled "Schmerz" which is the German word for pain. At that enlightened moment, we discovered that our guide could speak German. Not English, but German. We proceeded to communicate in a fractured version of the German language.

"Could I have acupuncture and end the pain immediately?"

"Nein."

"Why not?"

A shrug of the shoulders is the same in any language.

There was nothing to do but wait until the X-ray was developed. Tension mounted as the minutes ticked by. When the doctor appeared, he wore a smile. His diagnosis went the circuitous route of languages: Chinese to German (nicht gebrochen) to English (not broken.) Our sighs of relief and shouts of delight could be heard all the way south to Canton. For three weeks I hobbled around China with a cane, a swollen left foot, and a lot of pain.

For the remainder of the tour of this fascinating country, I kept the bus driver company as I observed Chinese culture from my seat on the bus while the rest of the group toured factories, shops, landmarks and other points of interest. If only we could have spoken the same language, the bus driver and I could have exchanged life stories and possibly formed a lifelong friendship.

I peeked at the life in the heart of that ancient country as I watched the daily routine of the people at work. How astounding to see a small, lean man, his muscles taut and hard from their daily Tai Chi exercises, straining to pull a huge load of freshly-butchered carcasses ready for the meat market. A small boy trudging at his side, learning what might well become his trade for life. Like all tourists, I took a lot of pictures and these photos taken through the glass of the rear window of the bus are now my most prized possession.

New sights and sounds rushed in on me almost too fast to record them in my mind. It was indeed a strange and different culture, so vastly contrasting the American way. It was astounding to watch four men tugging, pushing and pulling to move an enormous wagonload of hay across a cobbled street. No trucks, no fork lifts, no high powered machinery here — just muscles.

The Chinese people used the strength of their lean bodies to pedal bicycles, pull rickshaws and haul cargo.

The traffic pattern was equally astonishing. There were relatively few cars on the road, but thousands of men and women on bicycles thronged through the streets in a wide band, weaving in and out, creating their own momentum, barely making way for our tourist bus to pass.

Like all good things, the tour ended way too soon, and along with my luggage, I carried with me my impressions and thoughts of my adventure on another continent which I would sort out and muse over for a long time

The seventeen-hour flight back home gave me the opportunity to reflect on the wonderful trip and speculate on the future. I was just a bit apprehensive. What projects should I plan? What would I have to do to heal this silly foot? How long would I be off my feet? I wondered what Wayne was going to say when he'd see me limping along on a swollen, sprained ankle, leaning heavily on my exotic Chinese cane.

Our married life never was humdrum, so why start now?

At that time I had no inkling of what the future held in store for me. But I figured that if life's surprises came on an audio tape, it would start out with God's voice saying: "Testing, testing, testing."

If I thought for a single moment that we had already completed our periods of "testing, testing, testing," circumstances would prove me all wrong. That only happens when life is over. As long as we draw a breath, life is waiting in all its shapes and forms, and the real tests are still looming in the dense shadows of the future.

October, 1983
Weak feeling in left leg present at the time of my fall in China. Sprained ankle took four months to heal.

The next four months were rather trying, and I was often slightly annoyed with my ankle which took forever to heal. As it turned out I would have to wait almost 16 weeks before my foot returned to normal. I hobbled around the house, gave up my walks with Wayne and put my golf game on hold.

During the slow recuperation, I read a a lot, and every once in a while regarded my thickly bandaged foot with great annoyance. How a simple twist of fate — or foot — could have so immobilized me. I managed to cook our traditional Thanksgiving dinner and we celebrated the day with our daughter Judy and our grandchildren.

Before the turkey bones were picked clean, Christmas rushed in and Wayne and I prepared for the holiday season. Fortunately, I had done most of my Christmas shopping in China, and I didn't have to fight the crowds on one good foot. As I wrapped each gift, I relived my adventure, recalled where and when I picked up each trinket, and marveled how traveling the globe enlarged my world and expanded my mind. I wanted to do much more of that.

January was wet and cold, and I went back to my books and my writing. The days were brightened by visits from friends and neighbors, and the fact that one could play bridge sitting down. I welcomed every interruption of those long, dark wintry days with great enthusiasm, and was grateful for the friendly faces that helped ease my discomfort.

In spite of the nasty weather the pink camellia bush next to our patio had burst out into a profusion of delicate pink blooms, and other plants were gingerly poking tender green shoots through the dark, moist earth. When winter comes — spring indeed is never far behind.

By February the thick ace bandages finally came off my poor ankle, and although I felt not too sure about my left leg holding out, we followed through with our plans to spend the next two months in Arizona, as we had done for several years. We were looking forward to catching up with several of our good friends, as well as claiming our share of blue desert skies and sunshine.

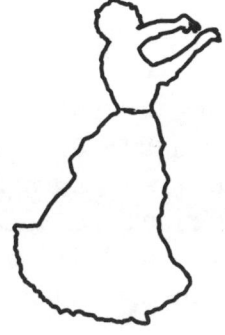

Chapter Three

Life is difficult. Face it and get on with it.
— M. Scott Peck - *The Road Less Traveled.*

February/March, 1984 - Sun City West, Arizona.
I discovered muscle weakness also on my right side. The middle finger of right hand not controllable. I am bothered by an unknown, nagging fear.

Each year, Wayne and I looked forward to our annual stay in Arizona with great anticipation. We had an apartment rented for February and March, and could hardly wait to see those friends from Nebraska and Colorado.

As always, we had a wonderful time. Each day seemed perfect. We golfed, shopped, danced, played bridge, lunched in Scottsdale, had dinner at the Camelback Inn, and attended the annual breakfast for 50 relatives, friends and strays. The White Mountains provided the perfect setting for our big morning cookout. We used up a ton of food, and talked on and on about the impressive consumption of 13 dozen eggs, 12 pounds of bacon, 120 rolls and countless gallons of strong, rich coffee.

One morning, as I was brushing my teeth, I noticed my right middle finger was floppy and failed to respond to a simple command to straighten out. Now I had two fingers that looked perfectly normal but were lifeless and unable to function. There was still the problem with my left foot which may have repaired itself from the sprain, but had not recovered its normal strength.

I tried to stay objective and stay almost uninvolved — as if this were a common thing happening to someone else. But as casual as I may have viewed my condition proclaiming divine indifference, I had become painfully aware of a general weakening of the muscles throughout my body. Ignoring my condition had not made it disappear.

I looked in the mirror, saw the raw, stark fear in my eyes staring back at me, and I felt a mighty hand tightening my stomach into a hard knot. My usual equanimity was out the window. I was terrified.

What gives? What is this?

Something was wrong. Really wrong — terribly wrong.

I conducted a guided tour of mental acrobatics which led to a variety of self examinations which in turn led to an equal number of self diagnoses. I went the route of per-hapses....perhaps I had walked too long.....too far....not long enough...had the wrong shoes....heels too low...too high...carried my golf bag too long, too far...too many heavy grocery bags...too heavy...the babies...I washed windows...stretched...reached...held...On and on I went trying to outsmart my body's troubled signals.

I finally decided I did not have enough body-building activities, my muscles needed strengthening, and the best way to accomplish that was to map out an effective exercise program. We had easy access to a gym, and I started to work out on a stationary bicycle till my face turned a bright shade of red, and I was huffing and puffing like a steam engine going uphill.

    I walked around the track for miles and used a stairstepper to strengthen my legs. I never missed a water aerobics class to exercise those lazy muscles, and turned into a regular exercise freak. It certainly didn't hurt. But, it didn't help either.

    Although I made every effort to enjoy the remaining days of our Arizona stay, willing my thoughts away from the problem, a restless uneasiness constantly hovered over me like Damocles' sword.

    We returned to Oregon at the end of March where spring was holding court amidst a profusion of blossoms that reached from orchards to shrubs, climbed trees and scattered its generosity on flower beds everywhere. A blazing maze of colors glowed against the shades of tender, green leaves and brightened the still cool and often mist-covered days. Nature had triumphantly marched over the drab remains of the winter landscape bringing new life to the earth. Perhaps my days of winter would end too, and nature would magically restore and renew my tired muscles and make my body blossom with strength and vigor.

    As inspiring and positive as these thoughts may have been, I also knew I had to do what lay at hand — go see a doctor and find out what the medical profession had to say about my condition. As scary as it was to live with fear in the dark hallways of the unknown, it is equally terrifying to look for answers — answers that may add to our terror.

April, 1984
I have started my parade of doctors and tests. I am scared — scared to death. Frightened that I have a disease that will take away my ability to walk and use my hands.

I made an appointment with our family doctor who insisted I see a neurologist immediately.

At once, without delay, he recommended.

We were able to get an appointment with Dr. Y the following morning.

After the usual check-in ceremony of filling out forms with a reluctant and tired ballpoint pen was completed, I was ushered through one of the many doors into an examination room. I was instructed to lay flat on a table and then the nurse-assistant hitched me up to a maze of wires and suction cups, the likes of which I had never seen.

"We are doing an electromyogram which is a process that measures the strength of muscles activated by nerves," Dr. Y explained in a business-like manner. He seemed to be in a hurry.

I gathered from his impersonal comments that a diagnosis would be determined through the process of eliminating a variety of conditions since he wasn't sure what he was looking for.

The next step was to take a myelogram to rule out any obstructions in the spinal area. It was intriguing to be able to watch my innards in action on a television screen — however I would not rate it among the top 10 shows of the week. My moment of intrigue and curiosity was cut short by a vicious attack of nausea and heaves that lasted into the next day. I vomited all night long and wanted to expire right then and there, but no such luck.

Next step on the ladder to reaching answers was a muscle biopsy, which was performed on my left arm.

Result: normal.

A blood sugar level test also proved normal, in spite of drinking a quart of liquid laced with artificial orange flavor — choice of the month — vile enough to make anybody nauseous.

Dr. Y couldn't think of any other tests to perform, called it quits and referred me and the results of the examination to another neurologist, Dr. Z for a second opinion.

I saw Dr. Z only briefly, and my visit with him remained a blur. He confirmed the findings — or lack of — rendered by Dr. Y. Both physicians were marching to the same drummer; I was the one out of step. However, I was told it would be a week for both physicians to complete their findings. I would be informed of the results.

May, 1984 - Final Diagnosis

I have a whole week to fret and sweat before our appointment for consultation with the neurologists to hear test results. I'm running more scared than ever. Drumming up activities to keep busy - golf games and lunches with friends.

May 15, 1984 was a bright, sunny day with the fragrance of late spring filling the air. The rhododendrons were in full bloom; their huge clusters of brilliant pink and purple blossoms were at their best, competing for attention with the red and pink azaleas, and punctuated with the crisp lacy, white blossoms of the dogwood trees.

I stewed and stewed about just what those two physicians would come up with — what fancy name, if any, my weary muscles would rate. I was glad when the day finally arrived when Wayne and I were on our way to the neurologist. Dr. Y would have the results of the month-long tests, which would determine why my leg and arm muscles had weakened. We had reached the point where we accepted the fact that there was something not very right. Apprehension, with nerves taut as a wire, we left the bright sunshine as we entered the sterile, pale grey atmosphere of the doctor's office

Dr. Y, a youngish man, perhaps in his early forties, had a pleasant face and curly brown hair which contrasted sharply with his stark white coat. He was of the new breed of physicians who retained his impersonal attitude and jealously guarded against allowing any indication of human kindness to creep into his demeanor.

He greeted us with no more warmth than he had exhibited at our first meeting. Unceremoniously, and with the same passion a weather reporter ticks off the day's forecast, he said:

"You have ALS", his face calm, his eyes void of expression.

Wayne and I stared blankly at this man — this edifice of medical terminology.

In unison we blurted out, "What's that?"

"It's also known as Lou Gehrig's disease," he replied with a touch of regret in his voice.

Shock and numbness took over. Vaguely in the back of my mind flashed the picture of Lou Gehrig in a wheelchair, making an impassioned speech about some illness or other in the middle of a baseball field, surrounded by hundreds of admiring fans. Good heavens, I was in high school then, and that was almost 50 years ago.

My mind raced to find other points of references, but I could not recall anyone ever talking about Lou Gehrig's

Disease, nor had I ever heard any kind of publicity about it or been aware of research being done for that matter. I had seen no articles on the subject, saw neither posters nor donation boxes at cash registers, or heard of funds being raised for the cause. And, I certainly had never heard of the term, ALS. (Much later we learned those initials stood for Amyotrophic Lateral Sclerosis.)

There was a heavy, dead silence in the office while the doctor waited for the verdict to sink in, and for us to understand the seriousness of the diagnosis.

With a somewhat awkward and apologetic gesture, Dr. Y reached behind him and produced a box of tissues. Standard procedure. We ignored the offer.

Jumbled thoughts leap-frogged through my mind. *The guy is wrong. What does he know anyway. Even though he relied on his colleague's confirming opinion, they are both wrong. All I have is a few weak muscles. No pain. So what's the big deal?*

Even though the vision of a wheel chair stuck like a leech in my mind's eye, I could not bring myself to ask the terrifying question, "Will I be in a wheelchair?" Nosirree. Sitting in that office with all the neatly framed certificates attesting to his medical savvy hanging on the walls, I was not about to ask that question.

Being confined to a wheelchair would mean giving up everything — golf, dancing, walking, strolling the beach, keeping house — the list didn't end. What about my hands, my arms? Would I be able to hold things, take care of myself, or what? Nobody, but nobody, was going to tell me I would have to give up life as I knew it.

Just in case that lump in my throat would not dissolve and would turn to tears, I dug furiously through my purse for tissues, while Wayne asked the doctor if he had some articles, bulletins, medical reports — any kind of printed materials — on ALS available. Dr. Y asked his receptionist to look for the appropriate information, but offered no further prognosis, or details of the disease.

The young woman shuffled through her files in the outer office and came up empty handed. Zilch. We were kept in the dark about what we could expect in the future and had no inkling of where to get information. How could I have a disease about which no one seemed to know anything except for diagnosing it?

Dr. Y offered no further commentary and I didn't say anything either. Perhaps he would have answered our questions, but at that moment, we were too stunned to ask.

We left the office and drove home in silence. I marveled at the fact that the sun was still shining, that the rhododendrons and azaleas were just as brilliant as earlier that day. The deep green of the mature pine trees formed an appealing backdrop for the soft-hued green of the new growth on the shade trees whose bare wintry branches had responded to the call of nature. How could everything be the same when this grey, gloomy thing, this mystery disease threatened my very existence? Didn't this golden day know nothing would ever be the same for me?

As in a tennis match, my thoughts bounced back and forth between doubt and acceptance, true and false, hope and despair, belief and doubt.

I finally settled in the comfort zone of my opinion that the neurologist was exaggerating. He was simply overreacting. He was way off!

However, as much as I talked to myself, as much as I denied the possibility that two physicians had to be right, deep down I knew this was not true. I wanted to crawl in a hole but there wasn't one big enough to accommodate me.

I barely noticed when we drove up to the house, shook myself into motion, got out of the car while Wayne opened the garage door. I went ahead into the house. Our comfortable living room, with its adjoining dining area that offered a glimpse, through one corner of our cozy kitchen, of the flower-filled patio, was bathed in the brightness of this sunny day in May.

But I didn't see it. I saw none of it.

I looked at the walls and saw a prison. I looked at the cozy couch and chairs circling the fireplace, and saw an army of wheelchairs challenging me. Where there was light, I saw dark.

When Wayne came into the room, we finally started to talk and decided to let our two children, Larry and Judy, know what we were facing. We called our son in Wisconsin and our daughter in Albany, Oregon.

I had not planned on my quavering voice, the tears and my choking at the words. Utter silence seemed my only refuge. All the courage I ever thought I had went right down the pike. Level-headed Wayne took over the conversation until I could collect myself.

I had previously discussed my concerns with my children as things had started to go wrong with my body, and apparently — their minds no less inquisitive than that of their mother's — had done a little sleuthing on their own. They had checked here and there and apparently had been more successful about gathering information on my condition than I had, but had kept it to themselves. When we dropped the big word ALS - Lou Gehrig's Disease disease on them, they already had compared their findings and had arrived at their own conclusions. I only confirmed their worst fears.

During those two phone calls, I learned more from my

children's simple research then I had from my doctors.

As we consoled each other, there seemed to be an overtone of hope — of maybe-it-won't-be-true, maybe-it-isn't-that-bad, after all it-could-be-something-else ... maybe ... in our voices.

When I hung up from our talk with the children, I pulled myself together, sought solace in the mundane day-to-day chores, fled into my kitchen and started rattling pots and pans, making a big thing out of dinner preparations. Maybe if I kept busy enough, I wouldn't have time for wheelchairs. I could be the first case in the history of ALS to be cured. Or, what? My Walter Mitty dreams were as useless as the two fingers on my hands.

We spent a quiet evening retreating deeply into our own thoughts which were laced with worries, fears, concerns and whatever else. Even though Wayne was quite composed, I knew this had hit him as hard as it had me.

What next, I wondered?

Well, life has a way of going on. From sunrise to sunset, ad infinitum, it charges ahead, and we follow the path that has been prepared for us. Given time and rising to the challenge, I would figure out some way to turn this negative situation into a positive one. I would not give in or give up.

I continued asking question about Lou Gehrig's disease and finally came across the information that there was an ALS Foundation in California. I placed a call to their offices and I was told that literature regarding ALS was indeed available, and, yes, they would send it to me.

I hate being kept in the dark about anything, and I was particularly anxious to learn something about my condition — after all, l had to live with it. Not long after that, I learned about the Muscular Dystrophy Association, and the wonderful work they did. In the years to come they would be my greatest ally in my battle with ALS. MDA helped with information and provided equipment which made my life easier and more normal for myself, my family as well as for my caregivers.

At that point, we continued to see friends and relatives and since my condition had become more noticeable, there was no need to hem and haw around. We told them our bad news. They could see that I walked differently, was thrown off balance easily, and that two of my fingers flopped around like two wet noodles. When we explained the characteristics of ALS to them, the puzzled looks on their faces gave way to downright disbelief, shock and horror, tempered with sadness. After all, most of them had never heard of ALS, and now they were forced to accept it as a threat to someone they loved.

Returning to our daily routine was comforting. Two months before we knew what we'd be facing, Wayne and I had mapped out an extensive automobile trip that would take us through Wisconsin, Nebraska and Illinois to visit relatives and friends, as well as a side trip to Yellowstone Park. I always wanted to see Old Faithful shoot up to the sky right on the minute of her scheduled appearance and get a look at the mighty Tetons. This trip was just what we needed to get away from ourselves.

We planned to be gone six weeks. I looked forward to traveling and perked up at the very thought of the trip. I must have been born with wheels in my genes. We put the house in order, packed our bags and went on the road. I wanted to travel light and leave my problems at home; or so I thought.

I still had not received the information I had requested from the ALS Foundation. I called them again and asked them to send the material along to our son's address.

First stop on our trip was Wisconsin where Larry Riggs and his family lived. Naturally the conversation turned to the subject of ALS. Larry opened his slightly outdated medical book to the skimpy paragraphs with its heading, "Amyotrophic Lateral Sclerosis." Hesitating, eyes serious and troubled, he handed me the open book. My eyes moved slowly over the few lines of type in order not to overlook even one significant word. One devastating sentence jumped out at me and struck me like the blow of a hammer — its prophetic message shattered what was left of my spirit.

"Patients with ALS usually die within two to five years."

I had not heard that one before.

Irrational thoughts somersaulted in my mind: *That can't be true. I'm only 65 and I feel fine. I have much I want to do before I die and, besides, dying only happens to old people.*

Suddenly the reality we were trying to escape raised its ugly head above the pleasures of the trip. A bolt of lightening cracked out of the darkness of the shadows surrounding me and turned the glowing embers of the fear in my heart into roaring flames of terror. What a future, what a sentence. Would I fit the two-year, three-year or four-year category? Or, would I make it to five years? What a sentence!

In the privacy of our room, I stretched out my legs in front of me extended my arms first to the side then brought them around so that I could look at them. Everything looked just fine, my limbs looked just like they always had looked. What was that insidious, invisible force that worked beneath my skin and out of my reach that was out to destroy the muscles in my arms and legs? Had the disease slumbered in my genes from the first moment of my being? If so, then what did I do to waken the sleeping monster? How...? When....? Why...?

I had no answers, and, it appeared no one else had any either — certainly not the doctors. Whatever it was I would be able to learn would have to be from people like me, ALS victims in perhaps more advanced stages. I turned away from ME and shut off the whirring blades of the windmills of my mind..

In the circle of my loving family, we resolved not to let anything spoil this visit with our grandchildren. We wanted to make sure our stay would be carefree and pleasant and would convert into a happy memory for everybody.

We played with the youngsters, went here and there and everywhere, and enjoyed the moment. One evening, we all went for a long walk — with one of the kids skipping happily alongside, the other blasting away on roller skates well ahead, all of us chattering about this and that. Even though I was contributing to the chatter, my mind was on other matters.

Like a dog with a favorite old bone, my mind kept gnawing on my worries — my fears, my doubts and the uncertainties of the future. Is it possible that in the future I won't be able to do a simple thing like walking? Perish the thought and treasure the present, I admonished sternly.

So engrossed with myself was I, that I never gave a thought to the fact that nobody had a guarantee the future would hold just roses, rainbows and chocolates. Everyone around me walked blindfolded into tomorrow not knowing what it would bring. Few have a crystal ball for accurately previewing events not yet born.

I believe that we all get our share in life of a little of this, and some of that. A friend of mine reflected that "We all carry our bundle, and we all walk in the sunshine and sometimes in the shadow." The only thing that was different for me, was that my blindfold had slipped and I could see a little of the future out of the corner of one eye — I had more than an inkling of what to expect.

In the years to come, and with endless opportunities to practice, I was to become a master of the art of banishing negative thoughts and relishing whatever the moment had to offer. When you know that your fate might not only limit your ability to move, to do things for yourself and others, but would eventually rob you of your breath of life, the present becomes doubly precious.

However, the idea of bad-times-to-come kept on lurking in the background of the most peaceful moment, ready to pounce. As much as I could, I kept the wild beast at bay during our trip. But everybody wanted to know all about ALS, and every time I talked about it I burst into tears. I was forever sobbing.

We made the rounds in Illinois and Nebraska, and spent a lot of time in the homes of friends and relatives where every meal was a family affair. With the help of all those dear people, I somehow managed to turn my problems into challenges — something concrete to handle.

We also visited my old homestead in West Point, Nebraska where I grew up. I loved going there since I had nothing but fond memories of my childhood, and still knew every inch and corner of that old place. The house looked the same. The upstairs bedrooms were still as hot as an oven in July, and probably ice cold in the winter. The wind still blew like crazy and the weather was hot and humid. Having become "cool" Oregonians, we simply melted.

In spite of the summer heat, I remembered the cold, cold winter nights. We slept in the upstairs bedrooms, and when the temperature dipped below zero we would snuggle deeper into the feather comforter mother had made. Through the years of butchering ducks, geese and chickens to feed our family of seven, she had saved the downy breast feathers and made them into warm comforters we called feather beds. Snow covered the farm and the land around it most of the winter, making the scene picture perfect, but not without adding to the problems of caring for livestock and chickens in the below zero temperatures.

Coming back to the hot summer day, I sat in the shade on the very spot where I played "tea party" as a little girl. I would plead with my older sisters to play with me, using my set of tiny, blue enamel dishes which three generations of children have since enjoyed. I still have all the pieces which sit on a small lace-covered tea table in our dining room, complete with a spool doll, waiting to "pour." The problem was my older sisters always had more important things to do than play tea time with a pesky five-year-old kid.

I smiled to myself when I looked at the swing suspended from the century-old cottonwood, looking every bit the matriarch of the land, and thought of the hundreds of times I had sailed through the air on its narrow wooden seat. Where did that little girl go? What kind of fate had been "dumped" on her?

Thoughts like these were as useless as an empty water bottle in the Sahara desert. I'd better switch gears to the questions I could answer.

Our trip home was uneventful, and as much as we enjoyed being with old friends and family, it was wonderful being back in our own domain. The flowers in the garden were in their rich summer garb, the trees seemed to have grown taller while we were away, and the weather was just perfect.

A few days after our return, a big package arrived from the ALS Foundation. Finally! I had waited a long time to get my hands on some literature on ALS, and now that the bulky envelope sat in front of me, I wasn't so sure I wanted to know that much about my condition.

I carefully arranged the materials on the kitchen table and started to read. Years later it is still painful for me to go over the detailed, vivid descriptions of the various symptoms and stages of Lou Gehrig's disease. It was horrible.

I was terrified of what happened to people in the advanced stages of the disease. I discovered that ALS affects different people in different ways — but none was pretty.

Carefully, as if not to bruise the papers, or curl a corner, I put everything back into the envelope. I didn't want to have to think about it too often. I had things to do, places to go, and I had better save my energy for the moment. No use to get all worn out fretting about what hadn't happened yet, might never happen at all. What's that saying about slipping on a banana peel?

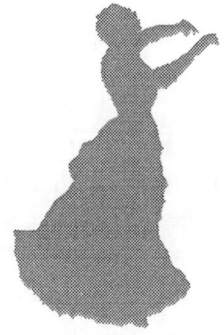

Chapter Four

You must do the things you think you cannot do.
Eleanor Roosevelt

July, 1984

It is now two months since I've been diagnosed with ALS. Some of my mental wounds have healed, my deep sadness is lessening. But the fear is always with me — the fear of losing control of hands and legs. I have not resigned myself to this yet and I have no intention of giving in without a good fight. Wayne's positive attitude helps.....I could not handle negative emotions at this point. His dependable self is always there — like a port in a storm.

I had played 18 holes of what I would loosely term a game of golf. Whenever I swung a club through the arc of the swing, my balance was about as steady as if I'd been walking on a tight rope, and I was afraid of toppling over. My score was proof of how poorly I played the game, and how it had deteriorated through loss of muscle power. There was no longer a doubt in my mind that the disease was advancing.

I was feeling completely dragged out and defeated, when Wayne appeared at the door wearing an ear-to-ear smile on his face.

"I've booked a cruise for us to Mexico," he said breathlessly, waiting for my reaction.

Well, you can bet your boots this made the day do a complete turnaround. For years we had casually discussed taking a cruise as something we would like to do sometime in the distant future. Wayne wisely decided this was it, this was the time. He had spent the morning with our travel agent looking at brochures, schedules and destinations. He settled on cruise with a November sailing date — just three months away.

What a wonderful surprise! I just glowed with pleasure and anticipation. Our spirits soared, we were flying high. These two Nebraska landlubbers were about to discover adventure on the high seas.

July 10, 1984

Appointment with neurologist brightens the picture. My type of ALS is slow-moving, gradually causing muscles in the hands, arms and legs to degenerate. At the present time it is not bulbar, which paralyzes the thoracic area, causing difficulty in breathing, swallowing.

My mind stopped racing and eased up on me a bit. I felt better about myself and life in general. I felt that time was on my side. However, it took several months for me to abolish my woe-is-me attitude. Whenever the demon of self pity showed its ugly face, I banished the monster by doing something pleasant. On the other hand, I could not wipe that Two-To-Five-Year life/death sentence from my mind that some judge had handed down in error to an innocent bystander of life. Tears always seemed to be near the surface.

July 12, 1984
Played 18 holes of golf. Not unduly tired.

What a game I played. What a story I had to tell about a golfer's dream-come-true moment. I'll always remember my 90-yard shot that went in the hole — the one and only Eagle I ever made. I can still feel the fluid motion of my six-iron striking the ball with the perfect rhythm that happens all too seldom, following through to perfection and seeing the ball bump the pin and drop in.

Maybe it was pure luck, maybe it was due to the fact that ALS forced me to slow down my swing. I have named the incident my Swan Song Shot.

Shortly after the event of that great shot, playing golf became a combination of ecstacy and agony: I was ecstatic when I did not feel wobbly and could strike the ball, if only for a short distance; I felt agony when I was in constant fear of losing my balance, and doubted my ability to control the trembling of my weakened legs. After 25 years of on-and-off golf, the time had come to give up the sport I loved so much. It was like losing an old friend. I stored my clubs, gave away my golf balls and made-believe it didn't bother me.

Of course it bothered me.

I continued to keep in touch with my fellow golfers, wrote the golf column for our local paper and served on telephone committees. I listened to my friends' golf stories, and cherished our friendship.

My golf days were over. Wayne and I had enjoyed many golfing vacations together, now circumstances brought change. (Oh,well, I thought, can't play golf on a cruise ship anyway.)

So be it.

July 24, 1984
Fasciculations (twitching) in muscles of both legs seem to be lessening and appear to have reached a plateau.

Fat chance. I was told later that the twitching does lessen after the nerves have already degenerated.

August 15, 1984
My legs are weakening and it's hard work to raise myself from sitting position. One year ago the first symptoms of ALS had appeared.

It is amazing what tricks the mind can play — how one minute my thoughts are flooded with deep despair and in the next moment my heart is light and joyful. The busier I was, the more I did, the less I worried and stewed. I stopped my gardening efforts but I was able to keep up with my housework. Cooking meals, baking cookies was a bit more difficult because I could not stay on my feet for more than ten minutes at a time before my legs began to tremble. I solved that problem by buying a tall kitchen stool, moved it up against the counter and did my food preparations sitting down.

AUGUST 27, 1984

My 65th birthday — spent with Judy and family at Black Butte, a wonderful resort, not far from home — I came to the realization I must appreciate the things I CAN do rather than bemoan the things I cannot do. We walked the beautiful hotel grounds and it came as a shock that I could not keep up with my family, and had to stop to rest often. Walking had always been a pleasure for me; now I was reduced to strolling, and I found the slower pace more enjoyable. In fact, I seemed to enjoy everything more. Sometimes life points its finger at us and it takes a shock to appreciate what we have.

At the end of summer Wayne and I joined some of our friends and attended a dinner dance at the club. I had a great time until I discovered that during a sprightly dance tune I dragged my left foot and didn't quite keep up with the beat. I wasn't "light" on my feet. However, the next tune had a slower tempo, and I had no problem following Wayne and the rhythm of the music.

I flipped the intruding feeling of momentary fear out of my mind with a quick toss of my head, denied what I had just experienced and proceeded to give the rest of the evening my fullest attention. I was aware that I had to guard against becoming paranoid about my condition and be constantly on alert for the slightest of signals or symptoms I encountered — or thought I encountered. After all, the mind does play tricks on us. Our imagination, especially when fueled by fear, can create phantoms with such accuracy that the monsters appear real.

Whenever I caught myself trapped by a black thought,

a woe-is-me attitude or an oh-my-God-what-next-terror, I stopped. I jettisoned my mind of negative ballast, dumped overboard anything that weighed me down and concentrated on the present. This was not a Pollyanna approach, far from it. It was simply living for the moment, the only moment we have and the only reality that exists. NOW.

Robert Frost said that "Yesterday is a bucket of ashes," and someone equally wise and nameless added "Tomorrow may never be."

I remember the words to a tune Wayne and I had danced to many times — a song of our days, "You've got to accentuate the positive, eliminate the negative..." I can still hear Bing Crosby croon his message over the airways.

Time is the healer and especially, when we stop digging in our wounds, the pain eases and the wounds close up slowly and heal. I began to feel better and decided it was high time I brought to life the things that had been vague and dreamy plans of mine.

For a short while I had thought my life was over, when it actually had only been the coming to an end of life as I knew it. I was simply beginning a new phase — and looking back at those years from where I sit today — that phase turned out to be more productive than I ever dreamed possible.

ALS — the monkey on my back — became the driving force that propelled me to tackle the things I had only considered doing *sometime. Sometime soon.* Well I didn't have sometime.

Sometime was now. If my muscle function was going to be limited, and eventually render me physically helpless as medical research-based information prophesied, I couldn't afford to wait.

I would write a book. At age 65, I was to learn how to

turn obstacles into opportunities, as well as learn to live for the moment — something I had not consciously done before. I suppose I was no different than the rest of humanity. We all act as if we'd live forever. We postpone and procrastinate, we ponder and wonder "just when we'd get to do that something that is so important to us" — and we sit back waiting for the right time, the right place, the right circumstances. And we wait.

I had run out of all the above.

I wanted to write about Wayne's and my childhood on our respective home farms in Nebraska. It would be a simple family chronicle that would recall the past and be a gift for our four grandchildren and their children's children. The past certainly contrasted strongly with the way most young people grow up now, and will probably sound "weird" decades from now. Hi-tech for us oldtimers meant a conversion from the kerosene lamp to an electric light bulb, a refrigerator and radio.

I settled back and let my memory go to work. Our Nebraska farm was homesteaded by my grandfather in 1857 — more than six decades before I was born, and I had heard the stories of hardship my pioneer ancestors experienced and the challenges they met face on.

I had wonderful recollections of my childhood. I remembered our family of nine gathering for supper around the large oil-cloth covered table, saying the evening prayer, and after supper reading by the dim light of the kerosene lamp. I thought about the delicious warmth of the old blue cook stove on icy-cold winter mornings and mother mixing yeast and flour in the huge crockery bowl with a blue stripe around the rim, used only for making bread.

She would place the dough in the warming oven to rise and when the yeasty dough peeked over the edge of the crock, mother punched it down and kneaded it vigorously. Sometimes she would let me be the first to poke the dough down with my small hand and see it deflate like a balloon when the air went out. The pungent smell of yeast filled the room, promising delicious golden loaves of bread or scrumptious coffee cake sprinkled with cinnamon and sugar. I could hardly wait to bite into these fresh-from-the-oven treats, which accompanied our noon dinner or our cozy four-o'clock lunch.

I recalled my favorite chore of gathering eggs and the excitement when I found a nest hidden in the hayloft of the old horse barn. There was always the danger of the brooding hen pecking at my hand as I reached under her soft warm feathers to retrieve the eggs, which heightened the adventurous dare-devil feeling of a little girl.

I would tell my grandchildren about pumping clear cool water from the well and bringing it into the house for kitchen use, when all they knew was turning on a faucet — hot or cold, please! Or what about a trip to the outhouse on cold winter days?

I would paint them a picture of the cozy warmth of cuddling into the soft featherbed at night, and describe the moment of shock as we shuddered in the below-zero cold when our sleep-warm feet hit the icy floor in the early morning and then hastily we picked up our clothes and scrambled downstairs. We were preceded by clouds of our steamy breath. We dressed by the warmth of the old blue cookstove. Father had started a fire in the early morning hours with corncobs and dry firewood which my older brothers had chopped, split and stacked in the fall.

Memories rushed in faster than I would be able to write them down, and I knew I had enough material to tell our story and document a way of life my children and their children's children would never experience. "Roughing" it during a night-out camping in the woods would be for them the closest thing to life on a farm in my days.

Memories into Memoirs was being born, but it would take two whole years to complete the process, mostly because the physical act of writing was painfully slow and I would encounter countless hurdles and obstacles in the process.

September, 1984
I tried typing today. Only my thumbs and a few of my fingers are functioning. Please, please, God, keep my fingers strong or how can I write? It is one of my great joys in life.

I have always been a competent typist, but when I attempted to use my typewriter, I found the strength in my fingers had diminished to the point where it was impossible for me to punch the keys. How could I write a letter, not to mention a book, without typing?

I was so discouraged and down that I literally gave up for a while and concentrated on things to do that seemed less frustrating. I just had to find a better way to write, a better way to accommodate my frustrations, and keep reminding myself that, "where there's a will, there's a way."

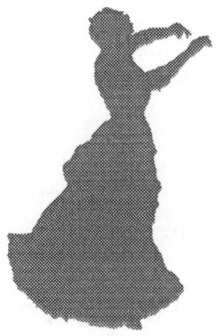

Chapter Five

> Fate keeps on happening.
> *Anita Loos*

September 30, 1984
I toodled around the golf course today in the electric golf cart watching my friends play. I would have rather played than watched, but it gave me a boost to be with friends outdoors in the nice fall weather. Legs disgustingly weak. Just happy to be out plugging away and not willing to give up so soon.

Raising above ... turning one's back on ... removing one's self from ... paying no attention to ... switching gears ... thinking of something pleasant ... calling a friend ... however you word it, not getting involved with one's condition is easier said than done, especially when there are constant niggling incidents that become the proverbial burr under the saddle.

There was always a reminder that things indeed were not right. There was that moment when all of a sudden a routine movement wasn't working. A glass went crashing to the floor when I couldn't grasp it firmly enough in my wimpy hand. Off went a Kleenex sailing through the air — the one I had sworn had been secure in my grasp.

The list was never-ending.

I was forever preaching to myself to "look at the bright side" — to look at what I could do rather than what I couldn't do. I was at it all the time (and still am) and sometimes I wondered how sincere I really was. Before I could answer that question, I got rid of it and pushed on. And, strange as it may have been, something nice always happened — a friend dropped in for a visit, the phone rang, a letter came in the mail, a rose bloomed in winter — something nice was always in the wings.

And if nothing else was happening, all I had to do is look out of the windows where nature in the guise of a splendid Indian Summer was blessing this land of ours with sunshine and colors. The whole world was dipped in late-summer blue and painted in shades of gold and hues of rusty reds.

Thank you world for this day.

October 9, 1984
I'm apprehensive about our three-day fishing trip on the Rogue River.

Much earlier in the year, Wayne had booked us for a three-day fishing trip on the beautiful Rogue River in southern Oregon during the month of October, and I was a bit worried just how I would be able to navigate the rugged banks of that wild river. Well, I would face the problem when I got there. We packed the car and drove off in the late fall sunshine.

I hadn't anticipated that the path to our cabin would be rocky and craggy and better fit for a mountain goat, than someone like me with wobbly, shaky legs. My problem may have bothered me, but it was of no concern to the two strong men who picked me up with ease and carried me over the rocks to our cabin. It was all so natural and no fuss was made. When it was time to do some serious fishing, our guide carefully helped me into the small boat.

Before we knew it, we were riding the rapids of the turbulent Rogue and were fishing for steelhead. We caught our share of fish, which our guides cooked over a crackling camp fire.

I was the greenhorn fisherman who won the pot for the first catch of the day, and later caught the largest steelhead. Fish don't care who is holding the line; they just go after the bait.

We had a wonderful time and not even the one day of skin-drenching rain ruined our holiday. It had been a wonderful experience — the kind that memories are made of.

October 23, 1984
I feel the degeneration of my muscles has worsened in the last couple of weeks. The two middle fingers of my right hand are flabbier, making it harder to grasp a glass or any object.

My limp fingers disturbed me enough to make an appointment with the neurologist. It was a waste of time. The man had little if anything to contribute. I would have to learn the hard way that "They" just didn't know a heck of a lot about Lou Gehrig's disease. With a feeling of desperation, I asked if a therapist would help me to retain the strength in those muscles which had not yet been affected by the disease. I reasoned that the stronger the muscles become the better they could resist the attacks to destroy them. Dr. Y said he would arrange it.

October 1984
In our search for more information about Lou Gehrig's disease we heard about a group support meeting for ALS patients sponsored by the Muscular Dystrophy Association. We gave it a try.

With the help of a city map, Wayne and I found the church in West Linn where the meetings were held. Using my cane — hesitating at the doorway — I walked into the meeting room, and headed for the circle of chairs in the middle of the room. We settled into our seats and looked around. Like children on the first day of school, we didn't know what to expect.

Our quick first glance brought us face to face with reality. We were shocked. Gathered in the circle were ALS patients exhibiting various stages of the degenerative effects of the disease.

Out of the approximately 20 people there were some who huddled in wheelchairs, several had lost the use of their legs and arms, one person was hooked onto a wheezing respirator, others were unable to speak. A few people, who were first-comers like me, clearly displayed their dismay, shock and disbelief at what they saw.

The person in charge began the meeting by having people introduce themselves. Spouses and caregivers gave a short report of the progression of the disease of those in their care which had occurred since the patient was diagnosed.

I was still in shock, appalled, scared, horrified and didn't believe for a moment, that I could possibly be affected in the same manner some time in the future.

Surely, whatever it was that went on in my body — the process which eventually would render me motionless, speechless and breathless — would have to be stopped.

I Was Not Going To End Up Like That! This was ridiculous!

Not Me — uh,uh!

I saw my disbelief and feelings reflected in Wayne's face. He didn't say a word, but I could see he felt the same way I did. He too denied the possibilities.

Things like that always happen to other people. Terrible things, catastrophes, disaster, misfortune, tragedies, fires, floods, life-threatening illness — all those things one hears about.

Not me — No, No!

In spite of our dismay and shock, we started to talk to people to get acquainted. With the common denominator of ALS, we quickly established a bond with the members of this special "circle of misery." We chatted about all sorts of things, knowing that we would see each other again and again. We would be able to see the changes in our bodies, compare notes, cheer each other up, console and comfort and commiserate as the disease would continue to take its toll.

We didn't know how often or how regularly we could attend these meetings, but felt certain we would go again. We went home depressed, yet somehow comforted knowing that we were not alone.

There are more like me out there.

The End Of October, 1984
This was a bad week. It rained constantly. The promise of the therapist appointment fizzled out because the doctor had neglected to make arrangements. I called our daughter, Judy, to meet me in Salem for lunch to lift my spirits.

Lunch with my daughter was fun. We skirted the most pressing subject of ME, talked about everything else but ... and I left glad to have one of my children close by.

November, 1984
This week is going very well.

The pattern of my see-sawing emotions should teach me not to give in to despair when things are difficult. In years to come I was to discover that when we think the worst was happening it was not so at all. Usually the picture brightened, even if only temporarily. Someone once said that if all the things we ever worried about had come true, we'd long be dead.

I thought about the prospect of our upcoming cruise, got excited, looked through my closet, decided on what I was going to take with me, and dreamt about tropical skies, ocean-blue waters and sun kissed white beaches. Sure felt better than worrying !

November 15, 1984
Two days before we are to set sail for Mexico ... we are not sure we're going. Wayne had a gall bladder attack. He always was one for the dramatics. The pain went away and our doctor decided he could

travel, bearing in mind my condition could worsen and we would not be able to go anywhere at a later date.

We picked up our flight on schedule and all of a sudden, we were aboard the Sitmar as planned — two people of questionable health. I had become firmly attached to my ornate Chinese cane, hoping my legs would hold out, while Wayne was concerned that his gallbladder might act up again. We should have learned by then that worrying is an exercise in futility, it ruins your day and life never happens on schedule anyway.

As it turned out, we managed to have a wonderful time.

The Sitmar was a magnificent ocean liner with a fabulous staff who pampered us with their excellent thoughtful service and wrapped us in luxury. We relished every minute of it.

When we made port and prepared to go ashore to see the sights, mild panic set in. How could I maneuver myself across the sloshing water into a tender which was constantly churning back and forth? It turned out to be quite simple. Two attendants picked me up and unceremoniously plunked me into a seat in the small boat which took us to the shopping area of Cabo San Lucas.

Quaint stalls with thatched roofs lined the waterfront, ready for the eager tourists to bid for the bargain of the century. Shopping in Mexico is an art which I thought I had perfected: select an article you like, ask Mucho? and proceed to exhibit a high level of reluctance at the vendor's exorbitant price. Then you delicately haggle back and forth until the vendor comes down to half his original price, which is twice what he expected to receive. I was ecstatic. I had just purchased a hand embroidered $25 blouse for $14. I could hardly keep the smug look off my face as I walked away with my prize package.

    I drifted off to the next stall to catch another so-called bargain when the man came charging through the mass of tourists, shouting, "Senora, wait." I turned around and wondered if I had broken a Mexican law. Maybe the man had decided it was too good a deal and wanted his merchandise back? No, not at all. In his hand he held my beautiful cane. "Lady, you forget your cane. I gif you fife dollar for it."

    I laughed and thanked him profusely. In the heat of the bargaining, triumphing over my clever purchasing tactics, I had left my cane and walked away unaided. Just the same, I was glad to have my faithful cane back in hand.

    The trip lived up to all our expectations and the time passed far too quickly. Each port was a picture of brilliant colors, exotic scenery, friendly people offering goods and crafts that bore the stamp of native customs and traditions. We loved the climate and the ambience of the tropical landscape — blue skies, bright sun and a warm ocean that shimmered between shades of deep green and midnight blue. Sleek white yachts and snow-white sails dotted the waters contrasting sharply with the color of sky and ocean.

    Life was wonderful and we made the most of it. After all, it would not always be a blue and golden world — not just for me but for everybody.

    That's life!

November, 1984

    Back to the real world after living a life of luxury. Wayne's gall bladder demanded attention again, and he had surgery. The operation was successful. The days returned to a level of sub-normalcy. A physical therapist gave me a set of exercises which I hoped would keep my healthy muscles in shape as well as strengthen them.

The holidays were just around the corner and we celebrated them in the circle of our small family, keeping things fairly simple to make it easier for me. Like last Christmas, I had done some shopping on our cruise and was able to avoid crowded malls and navigating the narrow isles in merchandise-laden stores.

Even though we saw our good friends in festive settings and had our share of Christmas cheer, the holidays seemed a bit quieter, a bit more subdued, and lacked a certain sparkle. Perhaps I had been imagining things. I was looking forward to something — I don't know what. Maybe I had been expecting a miracle at Christmas time — a cure for ALS wrapped in gold and silver under the tree. Maybe a Christmas card from my neurologist telling me it had all been a mistake.

It's only human to want what we want — Now!

New Years Eve, 1984
Goodbye and good riddance to 1984.

It may sound ungrateful to condemn a whole year and banish it from memory without a kind and gentle thought. But I was still teetering between the many uncertainties of living with a disease that promised, as sure as the sun rises and sets every day, to turn me into a helpless object of jellified muscles unable to lift a hand, to care for myself — unable to perform even the most basic physical functions behind closed doors and by myself.

I valiantly spoke about being positive, about acting

from strength and banishing weakness, but I had not as yet mastered the art of benign self deception to perfection. There were long moments when I considered my positive thoughts merely an act of blue smoke and I judged myself as being a practitioner of self delusion. I said to myself why would anyone get all excited about the "grand things" each day brings, when deep down I knew differently. I became a Dr. Jekyll and Mr. Hyde. I would be rosy of thought and peaceful of heart one day, and a down-in-the-dumps-poor-me-why-me the next.

I attempted to adjust to the reality that at some time in the future I would be immobile. I wouldn't be able to navigate under my own power. I wouldn't be able to move my limbs. I wouldn't be able to ... Stop!

During the month of December I noticed just how much the disease had progressed. It was indeed hard to ignore. I had to use my cane to get up or down the three steps in front of our house. I had to pace myself and rest often between simple activities. My legs refused to hold me up long enough to cook a one-course meal.

Visits from loving family members as well as dear friends popping in made it easier to maintain a positive outlook. A negative attitude drains the body of precious energy that can better be utilized for doing something important. Positive is the password of the day — every day. It is the key which opens the door to the impossible and makes it probable. I knew it in my heart, all I had to do was to live it.

February, 1985
I won't be able to dance much anymore. Is one of the great joys of my life about to be taken from me? I am alternating between deep despair and anger at this further degeneration.

The year had rolled around and in keeping with our plans, we packed our gear and journeyed to Arizona for our annual dose of sun, fun and golf, which we considered our personal escape from winter. We met with our faithful friends and even though they couldn't help but notice the change in my walk and the way I held things in my hands, they spared me their observations and I carried on as if...

We went to dinner one night where a band played some great dance music. Wayne led the way to the floor, and I had barely followed the beat of the familiar music for a few turns, when my left leg began to feel like it was made of wood, and I could barely drag it around.

We returned to our table when the awful truth hit me like a ton of bricks. I couldn't dance anymore. I excused myself and escaped to the powder room where I allowed myself a thorough but brief cry. Finally, I dried my eyes, pasted a smile on my face, returned to the table, and busily joined the animated conversation. No need to burden the people around me with my problems and make them feel uncomfortable with my tears and a pity-me attitude.

I would paste it on every mirror in the house. I would tattoo it on the back of my hand where I could see it. I would paint it on a windsock and let it fly in the air. I would imprint these simple words on my mind:

"Act happy and you'll be happy"

It worked most of the time.

I learned to make some weak excuses about not wanting to dance, but once in a while with the patient help of Wayne I managed to take a few turns around the dance floor to the beat of a slow tune.

What would I have to give up next?

When our winter holiday came to an end, I was looking forward to being "home" again. The security of one's permanent surroundings, the daily contact with friends and neighbors and the comfort of a familiar routine acted as a stabilizer for my emotions as well as for life in general.

I was glad to be going home.

March 21, 1985

After sunny and dry Arizona, we are back in beautiful Oregon, where we still marvel at its green serenity. Opening day of Charbonneau ladies golf season today.

I looked out at another spring making its appearance on the land which responded readily to the demands of the new season, undaunted by winter's memories. "It's not what life brings us, it's the manner in which we cope that makes the difference." Lack of a positive attitude causes feelings of depression and despair. I would not allow this to happen. When the monsters appeared at my doorstep uninvited, I would beat them down with my magic hammer and a few choice words. I would push the red "STOP" button and do something I enjoy - I would read a book, call a friend or have a chocolate.

Here it was late March already and my thoughts turned to the big event of the day — opening day for ladies golf. It was pouring rain. In spite of the bad weather, I wished I were out on the course. "I have to get used to the fact I won't be playing golf ever again. I must keep busy and find something to do in its place," I kept telling myself over and over again.

I sat down and made a mental list of what to do:

Maybe I'll get out my dried flower petals collected last summer and make decorative note paper for friends.

My photo album needs to be brought up to date.

I could make a separate album for each of our four grandchildren, including photos from when they were little and add their drawings which had graced our refrigerator a few years ago. This collection would make wonderful birthday gifts for them.

I could now do all those things I really enjoy which I had been too "busy" to do before.

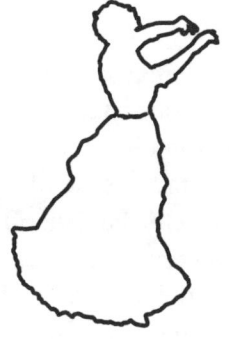

Chapter Six

Flowers grow out of dark moments.
Corita Kent

May 15, 1985
One year ago today, Wayne and I had been handed the diagnosis of my condition, to which I refer as the "final diagnosis." I'm still angry but I rarely cry anymore. I now have to use two canes and have stopped walking for pleasure simply because it is NOT a pleasure any longer.

I had lived with ALS for one year now and had made an uneasy peace with my condition. I went about each day living the best I could. I realized that there were people worse off than myself. I told myself the-man-who-had-no-shoes-and-met-the-man-who-had-no-feet story. Slowly I gained a new perspective and felt more at peace.

June, 1985
This is the year of the ramp.

Just like in all of nature, the changes in our bodies occur so subtly and secretly — behind our backs — that we can't notice them, until they manifest in either their incredibly mysterious ways of healing or, as in the case of ALS, in their vicious destruction of the body's mechanism. Our son Larry must have noticed the changes in me more than I had.

When he flew in for a much anticipated visit, he and Wayne put their heads together and decided that perhaps very soon I would not be able to negotiate the three steps at our front door, as well as the ones leading to the kitchen. I needed a ramp to come and go. Wayne and Larry built a ramp, intending it to look like part of the original plan of the house. They certainly succeeded.

Instead of just creating a ramp at each door, father and son built a gently sloping wooden walkway leading all the way to the street. Constructed from beautiful cedar slats that were masterfully fitted to each other, the new walk flowed gracefully between the new moss garden on one side and the patio and garage on the other. It was a lovely addition and enhanced the appearance of the approach to our home considerably.

When I looked at the leftover mounds of dirt in the courtyard piled against the north fence line, I saw it as a perfect chance to be my own landscape designer. With lots of help, we planted Irish moss and Scotch moss on the mounds of rich, dark soil, and soon two shades of green blended in the shape of miniature foothills. We had brought rocks back with us from our trip to the Snake River which we placed here and there between the mossy hills. The stones had been worn smooth by thousands of years of waters rushing over them, exposing in their structure the vibrant multicolored layers. We planted a lilac bush which brought back memories of my childhood when the fragrant purple blooms were the first indication that another long and cold Nebraska winter was on its way out.

The courtyard was beautiful and enforced my belief that something good comes of everything.

July, 1985
Unusually busy month. ALS is not hindering me.
Maybe I have reached a plateau.

Although keeping busy to stay happy was always on the agenda, sometimes we went overboard with activities. Wayne and I had planned a trip to Victoria, British Columbia with our Colorado friends, the Wardens, and saw no reason not to go. The highlight of the trip was to be a tour of the incredibly gorgeous and lush Butchard Gardens. The hour-long event brought on my first confrontation with a wheelchair.

"I can walk," I declared vehemently.

"Nonsense. Of course, you can walk, but it will be so much easier for you if we rent a chair," our friend Chuck insisted and remained firm.

A wheelchair it was.

What a strange feeling to place yourself into the hands of another person, to be pushed around in a "buggy" like a child.

In the first few moments I felt humiliated and conspicuous — then slowly, ever so slowly, I realized not one of the strolling tourists paid any attention to me. I was just one of the crowd. I relaxed and enjoyed the sights. The beautiful gardens coupled with Chuck's playful antics with the chair eased the situation. However I repeatedly addressed my companions insisting that "I can walk." I don't know anyone who is willing to relinquish independence. I was no different and would keep resisting for years to come.

July 30, 1985
ALS seems to be at a standstill. Is it possible that being busy and involved deter the progression?
Never underestimate the power of the mind. There is a theory that as the nerves deaden new sprouts form, take over and give the impression that a plateau was reached. Whatever works. Keeping in good spirits is the best remedy for any illness..

August 17, 1985
My legs are much weaker and I seem to have been in another decline during the past two weeks. What could have caused this sudden deterioration? Was it the pressure and fast pace of company and trips?

No sooner had I soothed my mind with the apparent fact that ALS and I most probably had reached a plateau, than I would have to re-address the problem and face reality. And, the brutal reality was the disease may slow down, it may stand still, but as sure as rain, it will progress.

This late summer day had been especially beautiful and clear, but it had also been a demanding day. Bathed in sunshine, under blue cloudless skies we journeyed through the magnificent Columbia Gorge, traversed the Hood River Valley, and ended up at snow-capped Mt. Hood. In spite of all the beauty on display the trip was long and tiring.

When we returned from our outing, I was exhausted and went straight to our bedroom to rest. All of a sudden my legs went out from under me and I found myself on the floor a few feet from my bed. I was shocked and stayed where I had fallen in stunned silence. Slowly I pulled myself into a kneeling position, and still on my knees, moved towards the bed. I pulled myself back up onto my wobbly legs and fell on the bed.

It wasn't easy to get some rest, I couldn't keep my mind still long enough to settle down. My thoughts whirled with visions of falling and flopping about like a beached sea creature. What if I fell in a store, on the street, getting to my car on a parking lot, in a restaurant? What if...what if?

Was this what the future would be like?

I finally dozed off and when I got up, my legs held me up, I felt fine and rejoined Wayne in the living room. The door to our bedroom had been closed and no one was any wiser as to what had just happened to me.

So be it.

I felt fine and a few days later opted for attending a dinner dance at the country club. I was having a wonderful time until I went on the dance floor. I couldn't even stay long enough on my feet to just sway to the music, let alone take one step to match the fast-paced tempo of the music. Slowly, and cautiously — praying not to fall flat on my face — I made my way back to the table. With a phony smile fixed securely on my face, I encouraged Wayne to look for a sturdier dance partner, sat back and watched him sail off across the dance floor.

I felt transplanted back to our high school dances, where the girls lined up against the wall of the gym hoping for some shy youth to brave the distance of polished floor that separated the sexes, and ask her to dance. Whenever I was not chosen and left standing against the wall, I felt forlorn and abandoned. That same feeling rose hotly in my throat and stayed with me. Wallflowers, we were called then.

I had become a wallflower. Permanently.

The music played on and I would never dance again.

I was so glad when the party was over, and in the privacy of our home, I fell apart. I cried and sobbed and cried until there were no tears left. I finally drifted off to sleep with the sound of the band in my ears with me sitting on the sidelines — a wallflower.

The sun rose bright on a deep blue August sky the next morning, and I was glad to be alive. I felt a lot better and gently, but sternly scolded myself.

"Come on old girl, get going. You can do other things. After all, when the music stops, you can keep on dancing to the tune in your heart."

I registered for the next creative writing class, and took a calligraphy course at the same time at the local high school, I read good books, wrote letters, talked to friends and made peace with life — at least a temporary armistice.

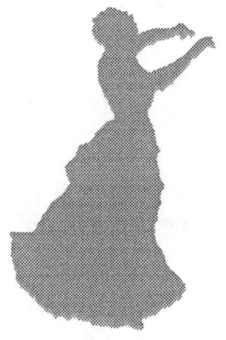

Chapter Seven

*You can either be a victim or a player in life.
Even though sometimes excruciatingly difficult —
it's lots more fun to be a player!*

October, 1985
I have been offered the opportunity to participate in finding a treatment for ALS. I have volunteered to be a part of a drug trial program in Kirkland, Washington.

There is a great deal of satisfaction in doing something to combat one's condition rather than to sit back and be overwhelmed by it all. The several letters I had sent to various doctors offering to take part in ALS research projects resulted in a reply from a Dr. Richard Smith of La Jolla, California. He planned to conduct a trial of the drug N-Acetyl Cysteine in Kirkland, Washington on ALS patients, and would I be interested? You bet I would. It was an emotionally difficult decision to make but Wayne's support and persistence gave me the final push.

We drove to Seattle and on to the neighboring community of Kirkland — sitting pretty on the shores of Lake Washington — and checked into a motel not far from the hospital.

I was excited when we took our places in one of the conference rooms at the hospital the next morning. Finally, I got to do something — something worthwhile.

There were 25 participants, men and women, eager to start the drug experiment, each one at different stages of the disease and all of them desperate to try anything. We were all grasping at straws. A look at them, offered me another glimpse of what my future might hold — truly a gloomy and depressing picture. Would I end up like this one? Or, like that one? Was I to be tossed into a future that held total muscle destruction in store for me? Would I turn into a limp, straggly chunk of hay being pitched over the side? Would I?

The initial evaluation session consisted of testing the strength of my muscles, (the test resembled a hand wrestling match) and reviewing my general health history. As I worked the muscle test, I was shocked at how much my muscles had deteriorated, how ineffectively my efforts as I pushed against the healthy arm of one of the attendants.

We broke for lunch and went to the cafeteria for a bite to eat. That's where we came face to face with some more of the crippling effects of the advanced stages of Lou Gehrig's disease. I had read all about it, I had seen some of the devastation in people at our ALS meetings, but the cafeteria offered one more look at human misery.

There was one person who had lost the ability to speak and made awkward guttural sounds in an attempt to communicate. A middle-age man was sitting at the table with his mouth agape. The thoracic area of his body had been affected. He was drooling and unable to feed himself. The muscles of his mouth no longer functioned.

The picture of that man — a bundle of helplessness — that portrait of silent indignity and suffering would never leave me. I put myself in his place. What will I do? What if?

The trial drug experiment seemed like a deep well from which to draw hope.

Out of 25 participants, eight ALS patients were selected and made the commitment to take twelve NAC capsules every day for eight months, not knowing whether it was the placebo or the real drug. I was delighted to be accepted, excited at the possibility of being part of a research program that might come up with some answers to this puzzling, dreadful disease.

The four-hour trip back home to Oregon was exhausting, but we were glad to have the first month's supply of capsules safely tucked away in our suitcase.

Once a month, for the next seven months we would travel to Kirkland where I was examined and where the next month's supply of NAC, or a harmless placebo, was waiting. Even though the trip was taxing, it offered a break in my routine.

The time just flew by and another set of holidays was about to happen. I had things to do and places to go. But I would have to do my chores a little slower and it would take me a little longer to get around.

November 18, 1985

So far I've taken 820 capsules of the trial drug. The excitement about this project has somehow waned, but Wayne sees to it that I do not miss taking those twelve pills daily. He is solid as a rock and his strength never seems to diminish.

I hope this batch of pills I'm taking is the place-

bo, because my legs have become weaker this last month. Maximum time for walking around the house is reduced to ten minutes before I am forced to rest. What a change in my life. After having witnessed the crippling effects in advanced ALS patients in Kirkland, I am filled with fear.

"That cannot possibly happen to me," I tell myself.

The time has come to acquire equipment to aid my weakening muscles. Through the Muscular Dystrophy Association we learned what was available. We purchased a lounge chair with an electrically raised seat, a raised toilet seat with handle bars, and a wheelchair.

Ah, yes. A wheelchair ...

I would have to get a wheelchair. I was told in no uncertain terms that it was a necessity and was assured the chair would be used only on certain occasions — such as shopping, a longer outing, a stroll in the park. How we are able to deceive ourselves. How easily we created a blue smoke screen around reality and then kept our fingers crossed and prayed that NOBODY would notice — especially not ourselves.

Just the same, I had progressed to a wheelchair because my muscles had regressed. Reality!

I stored the offending "wheels" out of sight, and finally brought them out when I needed to do some personal shopping. A good friend took me to the mall and I gave in to being pushed around in that "thing." I experienced the same out-of-control feeling I had the first time I sat in a wheelchair in Canada. I sincerely hoped I wouldn't meet anyone I knew. Just then four of my friends rounded the corner and almost collided with me. They were delighted to see me out and about, and no one paid any attention to my method of transportation. I realized my problem was in my head, not in my chair or in my physical condition. It was all in my head!

Other signs of the advancing deterioration of healthy muscle tissue were becoming evident. I had more and more trouble punching the keys on my typewriter and was reduced to using my knuckles because my fingers bent like tired reeds in the wind. I had talked with our son Larry about researching the purchase of a computer for me. I would just have to learn to use one of those new-fangled, hi-tech gadgets. I knew there would have to be a better method for me to do my writing.

In the meantime I would have to plug along and rely on growing and cultivating yet another patch of patience. I didn't care how things got done — just so they would get done. Necessity is the mother of invention, so "they" say, and I sure had the necessity and was ready to be inventive.

May 15, 1986

Two years after I was diagnosed with amyotrophic lateral sclerosis and 2,880 PILLS LATER, we are on our way to Kirkland for final evaluation of the drug experiment. Anti climax ... I already know what the research physician will tell me.

At long last the N-Acetyl Cysteine drug trial was over. Only two of the original eight participants were able to complete the experiment. One person had died, the other four had been forced to abandon the project for various reasons — one of which was the possibility they lost the ability to swallow, which is a symptom of the bulbar stage of ALS. At the onset, this symptom appears earlier in some patients, whereas others experience muscle loss only in arms, fingers and/or legs, as it was in my case.

Another possible reason for abandoning the project could have been the fact that the victims of ALS were discouraged over the failure of muscles to respond to the new medication. The continuous weakening of the throat muscles would make it harder and harder for them to swallow the daily dose of twelve capsules and promote a what's-the-use attitude.

The few survivors of the experiment sat around waiting to hear about the final results of the testing. We learned that all patients had been given the real drug for the first four months. The rationale was that if the drug were to slow the disease it would have to be effective immediately. The end results of the physician's testing showed no appreciable change and certainly not the slowing down we had hoped for. However, we all had the satisfaction of contributing to finding a cure for a terrible condition, if only by the process of elimination.

Having taken part in the research program made me feel better mentally, which automatically made for feeling better physically. Maybe it did something for everybody. At least we all knew that there were people working on finding a cure for ALS. So many diseases have been eliminated through the discovery of procedures and drugs. Who knows, ALS may be next to be given its walking papers.

On our monthly trips to Washington, we became acquainted with Dr. Patric Clapshaw, a research scientist who was in the process of setting up his ALS research laboratory. (As this book is being written, he is still fully dedicated to finding the cause and treatment for ALS.) In the last few years, research has been accelerated and renowned men throughout the world have been working on conquering this vicious disease. There will be an answer. One day!

May, 1986
Dr. Smith is beginning another drug trial. I cannot ... A different drug is being introduced, but I'm just not ready this time ...

I constantly reminded myself to keep looking at the positive and eliminate the negative. There is some good that comes of everything — a plus and minus exists in every situation. We may bemoan the loss of trees in a forest fire, yet it is the fire that clears the underbrush, makes room for new life to flourish and brings fresh growth to the forest. We run from the pelting streaks of rain, and hide from the roar of thunder, yet it is these activities which freshen the air and feed the earth. I remembered the words to an old Judy Collins song, "Something's lost, something's gained, living every day."

In spite of having been cursed with a killer disease, I had been blessed with the kind that progresses slowly.

And because of the unusually slow progression of ALS in my system, I have seen clinical trials and experiments come and go. There were drugs with long names that defied pronunciation so that everyone resorted to initials only, such as TRH. The drug had stringent side effects and for a time was believed to relieve symptoms. It never did.

New hope blossomed in my heart when Pergonal came on the scene. Scientists at Kirkland conducted a trial in July, 1987. The injections were $30 each and as it turned out were not a cure. I had my FSH blood level tested. Not significant. When it was thought that perhaps an excess of aluminum in the body might be a cause of ALS, I dashed off to our doctor to have a blood test for aluminum content. It proved normal. I was eager to rule out any possibility, as much for myself as for general research purposes.

Hope springs eternal, and I was certain that one day, there would be a cure. Maybe I would even be around to benefit from it.

July 10, 1986
I want to make every minute of this life count.

When I went through the pages of my journal I discovered that the subject which cropped up most frequently was family, and realized how strong our ties were, how important family was to us. Their lives mingled with ours; they were our extension and our future. Our two children and four grandchildren kept reinforcing our feelings of being cared for and needed. We always enjoyed taking care of our grandchildren when they visited with us for several days at a time when their parents took off by themselves. I remember some of the things during their visits that were memorable for us as well as for the youngsters.

When our grandson John was eight years old he came to stay at our house rather frequently during the summer. The attraction was not just his "Nana and Popup," but his grandfather's golf cart held a powerful fascination for him. He actually learned to drive it, and was consistently begging for an adult to accompany him. He handled the electric cart with care and caution, making his summer a special time.

As we watched the kids grow and change, and grow and change some more, we could measure time as they grew from baby to toddler to school kids. We were a typically proud and pleased set of grandparents and delighted in their presence. Kids kept things going, they never stood still and they taught us to look for adventure in the most common, everyday things. And I believe one can never have enough adventure in life. I shall never stop looking for it.

While I kept up my struggle with the results of diminishing muscle power, summer days turned swiftly into crisp fall mornings and cool nights. Winter came along too soon but brought the best Christmas ever. Larry arrived with my first computer and set it up for me. He patiently waltzed me through the preliminaries of getting to know that hi-tech marvel. There was a definite generation gap between me and my Macintosh, and it would take a long while before I knew how to work the basics.

I guess my generation is still working on understanding the principles of the toaster oven, and originated in the days when "bytes" were something you took out of a sandwich, and CD stood for cash deposit. But, ever since I learned that computers and their brilliant software were referred to as "artificial" intelligence, I lost some of my awe and narrowed the gap considerably. Also, I would never have been able to do my writing had it not been for my hi-tech wonder.

I plugged along working on *Memories into Memoirs,* and was so totally dedicated to the project that I even neglected my journal for months.

There came another "first" in my life which arrived in the form of a friendly househelper. I had always taken care of my housekeeping chores and it wasn't easy for me to let go and have someone else pick up after me. Later, a few years later, I would even have to turn myself over into the hands of a helper.

May 15, 1987
Spring is here again, and I have lived with ALS for three years now. I have adjusted mentally to my condition on a day-to day basis, but am filled with fear for the future.

Will I be able to cope with a mass of dead muscles? Will Wayne be able to cope? However, at this point I am grateful that I can walk. Using two canes is annoying to the point where I have a mental picture of flinging at least one of them across the room. I know it is only a minor aggravation which tends to overshadow the major issue.

No matter how much I worried about the future, I could not control it. The sooner I realized that the quicker I understood it, the better I would be able to enjoy what was at hand.

What was at hand — for all of us — is only the moment. Nothing more. Just the moment. Nobody realizes that until something drastic happens which puts gold in each minute. With that realization comes a boundless appreciation for the present, which adds an indescribable richness to the simplest things and chases away the clouds of fears and doubts about our life, our fate and the future.

The past is but a bucket of ashes, and tomorrow may never come. And, that places the moment on center stage, bathed fully in the spotlight of our attention.

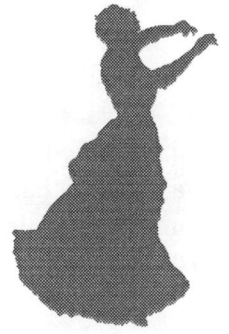

Chapter Eight

Life is rich and full
and I must make the most of the moment.

July, 1987
The effects of ALS are creeping up on me. I must type the final copy of Memories into Memoirs while I still have two fingers working for me. I am told there comes a time when one must stop rewriting a manuscript or it can be revised right unto its own death.

If ever there was a "creeping calamity," to put it mildly — ALS was it. It whittled away ever so slowly on healthy muscle tissue. With infinitesimal thoroughness it destroyed first one part of me, then mercilessly went on to the next. There was no "gradual" weakening — one moment I could use a finger — a blink of an eye later — and my finger went limp and useless.

Frustration and despair, fear and anger raged in a

kaleidoscope of garish, swirling colors in my mind, threatening to overrun the fragile wall I had been building — and reinforced daily — to shelter the simple pleasures each day offered. Slowly, I relaxed and the colors changed and softened until they harmonized with the warm glow that spread through my being when I thought of "my favorite things."

It worked every time. It was hard work. But it worked!

September, 12, 1987
We have attended a dozen or so ALS support group meetings by now, and we feel like old pros at the game. We contribute to these meetings with offerings from our bag of tricks and experiences — and we smile a lot.

I arrived at the last meeting of the support group leaning heavily on my walker. It had become hard work to drag one foot in front of the other — walking was going to be a major problem.

But then I looked around the circle as yellow pads and pencils were passed around with messages, answers to questions and bits of information scribbled hurriedly, and I felt lucky. I could talk. One pretty middle-age woman with a quick and easy spring in her step walked across the room to greet me.

"I wish I could walk like you," I said to her.

She whipped out her clip board and wrote, "I wish I could talk like you."

We looked at each other in mute understanding — eyes brimming over suspiciously — saying more than words could convey.

One young man, about 40 years old, a brilliant physicist, sent me a greeting from the confines of his wheelchair with the help of his voice synthesizer.

"Hello, Angela," the magic gadget spoke for him.

On the way home we always experienced the same set of mixed emotions. A strong feeling of sadness would come over us not just for me, but for all who were in the same boat. On the other hand, we felt good about the fact that we may have helped someone over a rough spot, made another one laugh — even though he couldn't make a sound — or lifted someone's spirit.

And, always in the background — much like an unwanted, disturbing and troublesome backseat driver — lurked the same nasty, nagging thought:

Where will I be ...?
When will I ....?
How will I ...?
Will I ...? and
Why ...?
Where are the answers?

I remembered the refrain of an old song: " The answer my friend, is written on the wind; the answer is written on the wind." Whoever wrote those words knew as much about "reason" and the future as I did. Nothing.

October, 1987

Just as I am feeling life is a real bummer and I'm down on my luck, along comes a phone call from a dear friend, Pat, inviting me to spend three days with her and golf friends at her beach house at the coast.

My, how that offer of two days on the beach lifted my spirit! It's all a matter of attitude, attitude, attitude. Pat's house was a comfortable place and we soon filled it with laughter and chatter. While my friends knocked themselves out playing in a golf tournament, I drove the car to the beach. I settled my back against a sun-warmed hunk of driftwood that some winter storm had tossed onto the sandy beach and spent hours listening to the soothing sound of the waves coming to shore. I marveled at the grey-blue beauty of the ocean, comparing its vastness to our insignificance on this earth. We are so small and our time on the planet doesn't last any longer than the flash of a firefly. Zap, and we're away to Eternity.

Born from feelings and reflections of a day spent in solitude drinking in the magnificence of the Pacific Ocean, words came to mind and took on form. When I returned home two days later, I plunked them out on my Mac, and recaptured my time on the beach and what was in my heart.

THE OCEAN
What emotions are awakened!
At first sight, wonder and awe
This blue-grey expanse
Reaching into infinity.
Slowly, peace steals into the soul.
The sound of the waves soothes.
It nourishes.
The vastness makes me feel insignificant.
Problems fall into place.
It is a healing elixir. ...
A soothing balm ...
A prayer.

December 16, 1987
 Today as I was working on my computer, I was shocked when I realized my left wrist was floppy. This was the first indication that the disease was creeping up my arm. I am distraught. Worried about what next. I must go on with writing my book and all the things I want to do yet with my life. Now.

I have had my Macintosh for almost one year now, and "Me and my Mac" have become quite friendly. I didn't think I would ever learn or use the vast range of the tricks it can do. But that was all right, I had no plans to turn into a computer buff any time soon.

Going over my notes and my journal entries, I realized how I skipped whole blocks of time where I did not comment on my daily life or on my condition. Perhaps I was attempting to lead a life void of interruptions from a killer disease. Perhaps I was just running away for a while.

May 7, 1988
 Today I broke my leg.

Of all the darndest things! I sat on my electric cart in the garage, trying to close the door, when I accidentally pushed the reverse shift while the wheel was turned at an angle. The cart took off, crashed and threw me onto the hard cement floor. I heard a bone crack — a sickening snapping sound, and a searing surge of pain raced up my leg. I didn't dare move, I knew I had broken a bone.

Petrified, I shouted for Wayne who was in the house. He must have heard the note of panic in my voice, and came dashing down the ramp to where I lay on the floor moaning in pain and muttering, "Oh shoot, now I've gone and done it!" Just what I needed, a broken bone.

Wayne called 911 on his portable phone and help arrived within minutes. Before I knew it, strong hands lifted me gently on to a stretcher and I was whisked away, all the while moaning and groaning.

Sure enough that leg needed fixing. Grumbling and full of pain, I settled into my hospital bed and got busy at restoring a sense of equanimity, settling down to work with the healing process and not against it. Ranting and raving, mumbling and grumbling wasn't going to contribute to my well being and certainly wouldn't do a darn thing for those around me.

Surgery was scheduled for the following day which, ironically, happened to be Mother's Day. This was the day for mothers to be served breakfast in bed. Well, I was in bed, but I doubted that I would get my tray before surgery. A broken leg on top of ALS made me wonder and speculate if I'd ever walk again. Only time would tell.

The operation went well, and in the following days my room became a garden of beautiful flowers in baskets and vases of all sizes. Dozens of cards arrived each day and the steadfast caring of Wayne and my family were my survival kit. All that love and attention certainly brightened my ordeal and lifted my spirit.

From the window in my pleasant hospital room, I had a view of a peaceful panorama where a thick fringe of tall pine trees curled against the distant hills to the east, softly outlined against a blue sky.

My mind vacillated between despair and hope. Up and down I rode my emotional roller coaster — hills of light and valleys of shadows; doubts and fears; complaints and gratitude. The spectrum of my emotions played on. I finally sorted out my thoughts and put them on paper.

WHY?

In my white-walled room filled with flowers
I seek answers.
Why is this?
Yes, limbs are weak
Hands fail to function
ALS has taken its toll.
Yet my spirit stands tall and shining.
Then
    the harsh jolt...
        the slashing pain...
           the shattered femur.
Is this a test of what the spirit can bear?
Is a mission yet undone? I know not
But
    I will conquer.
My heart beats brave and soars,
To reach to the skies
Love of family and friends pulls
    like a current
        surging toward courage ...
           serenity ... .joy!

On the fifth day my friendly, smiling therapist made moves toward getting me out of bed to put me on a built-up walker. I was horrified. Me? Out of bed? Cheerfully, the therapist ignored my anxiety and somehow I was elevated into an upright position.

Step right foot, slide left foot, be calm, be calm. I did this twice each day and then insisted on having a third walking session up to ten steps. I became less anxious as my walk improved.

The day I left the hospital the doctor cornered me and with a grin on his face confessed, "I never thought you would walk again, but you have proven me wrong."

His words gave me the strength I needed. In fact, I was almost exuberant. Sure, I would walk again and life would be "normal."

A bit reluctantly, I left the sheltered environment of the hospital where caring nurses and attendants had been at my beck and call. When I got on my feet at home, my walk was as faltering as a baby's first steps, but just the same, I was pleased with my efforts and proud of my accomplishment. Inner joy was the ray of light that chased the murky clouds of fear until they disappeared.

June 24, 1988

Joy, indeed! The therapist showed me how to get back into my three wheeler. After seven weeks, maybe my life could get back to some sort of normalcy.

To celebrate, Wayne took me out for an ice cream cone. Good kid!

We also went out to dinner and we were able to resume some of our former activities. Indeed, life is what you make it — color mine beautiful!

I came across the following passage from Rabbi Kushner's book, *When Bad Things Happen To Good People:* "The facts of life and death are neutral: We, by our responses, give suffering either positive or negative meaning. Illnesses, accidents, human tragedies kill people. But they do not necessarily kill life or faith."

I shall remember these words.

August 16, 1988

If nothing else, being afflicted with ALS has opened up new avenues in my life. A worker for Muscular Dystrophy called and asked me to appear on the Labor Day Telethon fund raiser. It was exciting and rewarding. I hoped it would help others living with the debilitating effects of a neuromuscular disease. It was just a brief shot of me in my wheelchair, while an announcer explained ALS to the television audience in an effort to make the public aware of the devastation of this complex disease.

October 27, 1988
Life goes on, and I am glad I am part of it.

We gave a "theatre" party for twenty-five friends to celebrate Wayne's honor of being inducted into the Athletic Hall of Fame, in the Peru (Nebraska) State College, his Alma Mater.

After dinner, our guests gathered in front of the television set — poor unsuspecting lambs. They never realized they would be obligated to watch a video of Wayne's "day in the sun," which expounded on his virtues as an athlete in the 1930s to the point where a stranger appearing on the scene might remove his hat, place it over his heart and bow his head, believing he was listening to a eulogy.

Wayne remained in the kitchen making popcorn during the "movie" — you can imagine whose idea it was to parade his fame before a willing group of friends.

Our grandson, John put the popcorn in small bags and served it to our guests to ease their pain. Everyone thought it was fun and they even prolonged the evening by asking to see the film made of his "Roast" which had been produced by Wayne's golfing buddies about that same time. One of his golf partners presented him with the following words:

WHEN ANGELS CRY

> If everyone, everywhere
> In this whole wide world
> was always as nice and decent
> As our man Riggs
> (Except when he misses two-foot putts)
> How splendid this world would be.
>
> And when to Heaven Wayne ascends
> And partner of God he becomes
> In golf above the skies
> Surely angels all will cringe
> When God and Wayne miss two-foot putts.

I had a great time and played the radiant hostess hobbling around on my walker, enjoying every minute of that special night.

It's just like the saying on one of my book markers: "Life is what thou maketh it … so maketh it fun."

Daily, I worked on looking at the bright side of life, counting my blessings and plugging along. That is not to say there weren't moments when I felt a bit foolish about playing ring-around-the-rosy when I couldn't even pick up a feather I dropped on the floor, when common-every-day activities no longer were part of my life. I would be a liar if I were to deny those feelings.

The days of summer must have had wings that year, and flew by in all their sun-warmed lightheartedness and took us swiftly into the next season. It reminded me of some old movie, and how film makers resorted to letting an off-camera wind blow the pages of a calendar into the air to demonstrate the passing of time. When I looked at the golden-brown leaves whirling on the ground being scattered and tossed meaninglessly about by a brisk fall breeze, they became the long past days of spring and summer from the calendar days of my life — brittle, fragile and robbed of the green lushness of their summer vigor.

Stop. Switch gears.

Grey thoughts are like clouds, they block the sunlight.

November 7, 1988

At this point my main concern is the gradual loss of power in my right hand. Writing letters by hand has become a thing of the past, and all of my personal correspondence will have to be done on my computer. I hope people will understand.

December, 1988

I have always been an avid bridge player, and I love the game. A new problem has come up. I haven't been able to shuffle, deal or hold my cards for quite some time, and have resorted to using a card holder. However, getting the cards into their slots is becoming more difficult all the time. Will I have to give up one more thing I enjoy?

I realized that I was not the only one on the face of this earth with a big problem. The saying goes that when one door is closed another will open. Quite a few doors have slammed shut on me already. But I kept jamming my foot in the door that led to a good game of bridge. That door would stay at least ajar, if not wide open. I wasn't ready to give up bridge because I desperately needed a social life, and I loved the game. So I fumbled through the mechanics of card playing, substituting my lack of finesse by trying to make brilliant bids, not always successfully.

Thanks to the slow progression of ALS in my case, five years elapsed before it became impossible for me to lift my hands to sort my cards, place them in a holder and play them. Friends offered to sit by my side and play my cards according to my instructions. Years later, I continue to play bridge — and as the song says, "Oh, I get by with a little help from my friends."

Each time a new challenge presented itself, a solution followed on its heels. With child-like glee, I was always so pleased with the solution, that I forgot the seriousness of the challenge. You can't help being stung by life, but you can find ways to take the bite out of the sting!

I had also come to the conclusion that one should not worry about things before they happen. What if I worried about something night and day and when it happened — I was out to lunch? There is a fine point between planning and preparing for the unknown and worrying about it.

Christmas, 1988

What could have been a happy holiday season turned out to be the beginning of an incredibly difficult period in Wayne's life. It was a nightmare. He had to be hospitalized and on Christmas Eve he underwent surgery for the removal of a tumor. On Christmas morning his thoughtful physician delivered him to our front doorstep complete with a red bow tied jauntily around his neck to match the festive mood of the day. We also received the diagnosis. It didn't have a red ribbon around it.

We added another dreaded terminology from the medical lexicon to our list of personal terrors — Wayne had cancer. On New Year's Eve the urologist removed a portion of his bladder. What a way to end the year. Throughout 1989, Wayne was in and out of the hospital so many times that people thought he had purchased a wing with the thought of making it his permanent home.

During these demanding times, my own condition became a secondary issue. However, it was brought back into focus when another experimental treatment came to my attention. L-Threonine, an amino acid, was believed to be effective in halting ALS symptoms. In desperation, I took the prescribed eight pills per day, plus vitamin B-Six which had been recommended by the researchers. After several months of popping pills, we had to agree that L-T was no quick cure for the disease — it was no cure at all.

Even though I knew from the onset that an experiment is just that — an experiment — there is always a let-down and a good case of disappointment when a bubble bursts. We bury our hopes and dreams along with another set of worn out, tired could-have-beens. Whatever the circumstances may be, the best anyone can do is explore all avenues and never give up.

If Wayne and I ever entertained the thought that we had been thoroughly tested in the past we were quite wrong. Yesterday's problems were child's play compared to what was yet to come. In the first six months of 1989 he was hospitalized time and time again. He underwent the removal of a cancerous bladder, had a pulmonary embolism and was treated for several serious bouts of infection. There was so little I could do for him, yet I relied so much on his being constantly at my side. The daily phone conversations with Larry, Judy and our grandkids, always brightened our days and kept me on an even keel.

I'm sure I would have hit the bottom of despair had it not been for our friends. Not a day went by without a friendly face dropping in for a cup of tea bearing a bunch of flowers, showing up with a batch of freshly-baked cookies, home-made casseroles, kind words of encouragement, and generous offers for taking me places. People are wonderful — they opened their arms and their hearts to me, and I walked right in.

July 30, 1989

Wayne's 74th Birthday. Considering the ordeals he has gone through, this day is indeed a special occasion — we celebrate life.

Judy, John, and Susan, arrived bearing wonderful gifts. They brought the birthday dinner — a whole, fresh salmon and Wayne's favorite dessert, two large lemon meringue pies. When the perfectly baked salmon — gills out, eyes turned to the ceiling — was brought to the table in all its glory, Judy placed seven and four candles into the salmon's belly, lighted them, and we joined in a rousing rendition of Happy Birthday To You. If we hadn't taken a picture of the scene, no one would have believed this odd and "fishy" ceremony.

It was probably the happiest of all birthdays. Life is still the most viable alternative and a happy heart is the frosting on the cake — in our case it was the frosting on the salmon!

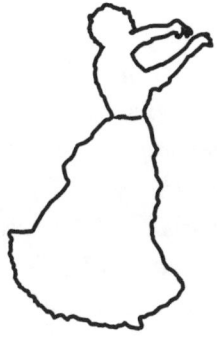

Chapter Nine

The greatest part of our happiness or our misery depends on our dispositions and not on our circumstances.
Martha Washington

August, 1989
"Memories into Memoirs" is completed.

Finally, I finished the book. Luckily, Larry and Lori were in town and with their help, we got the manuscript to the printers and later on to the bindery, where we chose a maroon hard cover with gold stamping. I would never have been able to accomplish this feat without their assistance. Fifty copies were printed, bound and mailed to grandchildren, nieces and nephews just in time for Christmas giving. The recipients' appreciative response for my efforts was all the reward I needed. I could truthfully say, "I did it and I'm glad."

October 8, 1989
Today is one of those glad-to-be-alive days. The weather is a perfect 75 degrees, bright sunshine enhances the brilliant fall colors on parade. As I ride in my Classy Chassis around the grounds, I am grateful for being independent and able to roam about on my own to enjoy this day. Back in the house, I write in my journal and some of the joy disappears when I bring up reality. My left forefinger is like a wet noodle. It is the one I use for typing. I may have to learn typing all over again.
Larry has reassured me there are computer aids if the time ever comes when I should need them.

November, 1989
Six years ago I walked the Great Wall of China. Today I shuffle along with snail-like pace leaning heavily on my walker, but am thankful I can at least still walk around the house — after a fashion.
I spent a great day at Shirley's house playing bridge with friends. Then why do I feel so defeated? I cannot rise up from a chair by myself. It takes two people to hoist me to a standing position; my dignity leaves me and I feel humiliated. I am glad I have the electric lift chair at home.

November 5, 1989
Since my ability to type with my fingers — like everybody else — has gone to pot, I keep devising new methods to work on the computer. Yesterday when I found my forefinger would not function I used the knuckle of my middle finger on the left hand

and thumb of my right hand. I have to keep on writing — I have an idea for a book.

Necessity is truly the mother of invention. After a while, I found that clutching a pencil between my fingers — eraser-end down — worked reasonably well for tapping out one letter at a time with the computer keyboard sitting on my lap. One letter at a time makes into a word — words make sentences — sentences make paragraphs, paragraphs fill pages, and pages make into a book.

I was writing a book one letter at a time — just like everybody else!

I have always been fascinated with genealogy — finding out where we come from; who went before us; who and what were our ancestors. I knew mine came from a small town in Germany, crossed the ocean and settled on the plains of Nebraska, where some members of my family still occupy the old homestead farmhouse.

I was going to tell their story so that they would live on and be remembered by the generations to come. Some people know little or nothing of their family's beginnings, and I wanted our grandchildren and their children to know their origin. Our ancestors left us a heritage of courage and ethics that will never go out of style — and the generations to come need to know about it.

I would have quite a bit of research to do. Just the thought of attacking another writing project added sparkle and excitement to my life. I have discovered that if you keep your mind busy with productive work, it won't have time to let your body know something's wrong!

I already had my "green" file loaded with bits and pieces of information on my family, but I needed more, and I ventured out to one of our local "new and used" booksellers for a look at the store's "Nebraska" section. With my son by my side, I cautiously cruised the narrow aisles of floor-to-ceiling book shelves, and whenever I spied a title that promised information, Larry dutifully piled the book on my lap.

By the time we got to the cash register, I could barely look above the musty pile of books I had collected on Nebraska. It would keep me busy for a while

November 15, 1989
I am pleased with myself. I have written the first chapter of my very own "Great American Novel." I think I'll call it "Voices of the Prairie."

I had begun a new adventure. I told myself that if I didn't start the book, I would never finish it. (It doesn't take a genius to understand that!) Letter by letter, word by word, and so on, my project took on shape, and the days just flew by.

November 27, 1989
Time out for a refreshing visit from granddaughter, Susan, which can be compared to having a whirlwind in the house.

Eight-year old Susan loved to play dress-up with me. She would rummage through my jewelry box and pick out her favorite pieces for both of us and head for the closet where I kept a box of old and "funny" stuff just for that purpose.

Susan decided we should dress up like elegant ladies, and take a walk in our finery. She found an old hat in the dress-up box, as well as my old mink cape and other "haute couture" items, and with a little help, we were ready to strut our stuff.

We "walked" up and down the lovely tree-shaded streets by our house on that sunny 90-degree day in great leisure. What a sight we must have been! Here I was in my Classy Chassis draped in that ratty, moth-eaten mink cape, clutching my granddaughter's favorite pal — a quite obese, stuffed pink pig. We were both drowning in gobs of jewelry, and she was pushing a toy duck that waddled from side to side. There's nothing like being with a little girl to become a child again.

December 13, 1989

Forever at my side, with the help of faithful Toni, Wayne and I prepare for Christmas. As I look at us, I realize we both are battling ALS. Wayne has been doing things around the house and for me that I never thought I would have him do. That was my job! I'm alarmed at the added weakness in my legs and find it difficult to walk from room to room, even with the support of my walker. I sort of shuffle from one place to another.

We were trying to adjust to an altered lifestyle. Wayne and I had switched roles. I didn't know there was so much to do every day, until I couldn't do it any more. Wayne shopped for groceries, ran errands and kept house. He did everything he used to do, plus most everything that had been my department. That's not how it had been, nor was it how we had planned our life of retirement!

It certainly couldn't have been easy for him, and I was always so glad when he was able to escape to the golf course. Like me, he loved the sport, the lovely setting of the greens, and the jovial company of his golf buddies. When he was out of the house, I just headed for my computer and spelled out a few words.

I wasn't much help with trimming the tree that year, or wrapping gifts or helping in the kitchen, but I made an excellent project manager, traffic cop and general activities director. Wayne carried the load and enjoyed all the goings on. Friends came bearing gifts and goodies, and the rounds of holiday parties in our little community kept us going from one festive home to the next. It was a joyful time — so different from last year. Thank God that was over; Wayne has recovered nicely and we survived. Indeed we had been tested, but that made us only a bit "testier," I guess. I also believe we have been blessed.

Christmas, 1989

Judy, John, and Susan arrived with two laundry baskets full of gifts, which practically overwhelmed our small table-top Christmas tree. With our family around us, we had a happy holiday, and forgot our problems. With the aid of our speaker telephone, we were able to talk to our Wisconsin children and have them with us in the room.

December 31, 1989

The decade of the 1980s is dying. According to medical statistics of people with ALS, I am supposed to be dying too. Having already passed the two-to-five-year prognosis, I feel there is a lot of living yet left for me.

Happy 1990!

Saying goodbye to a year, especially a whole

> decade, is a time to stop and think. I reflected on the many things for which I was thankful and briefly reviewed those events I could have gladly done without. The sages insisted that there's a reason for everything, and the Beatles told us, "There will be an answer ... let it be ..."

We were both alive and reasonably well, considering that Wayne had seven (or was it eight) hospital stays, which included three (or was it four) major surgeries. Looking back on the past year, I believed that heaven can wait. I am fortunate to have a wonderful husband of 47 years (who can actually cook, although sometimes under duress), as well as two outstanding children.

Our four grandchildren are compassionate and caring people — each one unique as fingerprints. We have lived in or traveled through all fifty states and have learned a lot about the world. We are blessed with fine friends who continue to add joy to our lives. We've come a long way but there is still more ahead.

> *January, 1990*
> *Just what I needed to start the new year — a case of shingles — thank you very much. I'm writing this at 2:30 in the morning while eating Fig Newtons. I feel miserable but my doctor assures me it's not terminal. It just feels that way.*

Somehow I had the notion that having ALS would exempt me from other more common nuisance illnesses. No such luck! I had shingles.

Nasty, narrow red welts and a screaming, red-hot pain encircled my waist. I couldn't fasten a skirt. I couldn't bear to have anything come in contact with the inflamed and excruciatingly painful area. What a nerve-wracking experience! How long was this going to last? I kept saying to myself, "I can't stand this another minute," but apparently, I could!

Wayne and I had been closing down his aunt's household after her recent death. Every day I wheeled over to her house, and every day I became more frustrated at my physical disability. There were more than 1001 items in her kitchen cupboards alone, and it took a visit from Judy and a dozen friends to fetch and carry and do the leg work.

I fretted over my job of having to make decisions on how to dispose of auntie's earthly goods which gave me a permanent knot in my stomach, and probably opened the door wide to let that case of the shingles walk in on me. No matter how I wailed and railed against my fate, I didn't change anything, the infection ran its course. I found brief moments of solace in the thought that "This Too Shall Pass! It all comes to pass," a Chinese sage exclaimed 500 years ago,"Nothing comes to stay!"

I realized how "outside" situations and events affect our "insides" — how those things we let disturb us, rankle and worry us, often manifest as a disease. The body is such a magical machine, and in spite of the great strides medicine has made, we still didn't understand what really went on to influence our cells to do wild and crazy things — like getting sick. Sometimes I also wondered if the real answers to the human condition would ever be found through hi-tech methods, scientific research in chrome and glass laboratories.

In the meantime, I learned to endure, and hired more help around the house.

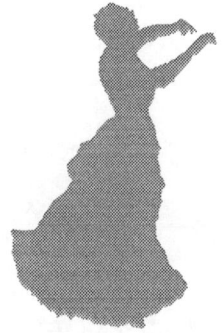

Chapter Ten

Bearing up under the load of living with an immobilizing
condition is like pushing a rope uphill.
One must keep trying, even though the greatest
effort doesn't stop the rope from dropping
right back in one's face.

Jan. 28, 1990

Once again seven-year-old Susan helped me regain perspective and brightened my day. Since we both loved tea parties, my granddaughter got out her set of small dishes and along with a batch of Oreo cookies we had a special party, pretending we were at high tea at the elegant Empress Hotel in picturesque Victoria, Canada.

I sat across the table from Susan and looked at her young and lively face as she informed me, "Here comes the waitress. You order first, grandma."

I looked in the direction of the phantom waitress and placed my order: "I would like hot tea, scones, and cucumber sandwiches."

It was Susan's turn, and without a moments hesitation she made her desires known: "I want a corn dog with ketchup and mayo on the side."

So much for class. A seven-year old has her own set of tastes.

April 22, 1990

It's very easy to lose heart when you have weakening muscles to contend with, along with the never ceasing hurt and itch syndrome of the shingles. In addition to all that, a gloomy fatigue spreads over me like a fast-growing fungus. I force myself to rest for a while and let my mind create new energy.

I discovered that fatigue is another staunch enemy of the ALS patient and that the course of progression of the disease is as unpredictable as rain. Fatigue appeared without fail and remained at my side — not the good tired feeling after having played a round of golf, jogged two miles, or danced all night — but the depressing deep distress that hovered dangerously close on the edge of despair. Fatigue and despair teamed up and created those black moments of the soul where no song can cheer you. Combining forces, they closed the door to the music of life and drew dark drapes across the windows that let in light for the heart.

The only cure I knew for the "tired, black howlies" was a good rest — it brightened the picture and lifted my spirit. Through it all, Wayne plugged along at my side with saintly patience, ever watchful and aware of my needs. I was truly blessed.

May 3, 1990

Never say die! Not only is spring here, but

Wayne is making reservations for a cruise to Alaska for the month of August. We are both looking forward to a change of scenery. Another adventure is waiting for us. I can handle that!

June 13, 1990
Today is our 48th wedding anniversary.

Two women much younger than I asked me for the secret of a long and happy marriage.
"Secret?" I asked, astonished. "It's no secret. Be tolerant of your mate, give more than you take, and hope that he is just as tolerant of you."
Perhaps that wasn't what they had expected to hear. Maybe it was too simple and not romantic enough. Whatever, they both looked a bit disappointed as they tried to digest my brief advice. All I know is that it had worked for us.
To celebrate we took our friends, Peg and Joe, to dinner, surrounded by balloons and slim glasses of sparkling champagne. Driving home in our red van (the one with the magic carpet ramp) we were treated to the most spectacular, colorful sunset Oregon had to offer — nature's personal greeting card to fit the occasion. We counted our blessings.
I had not been driving for quite a while and was surprised and somewhat pleased with myself that I did not resent the fact that I could no longer just pop in the car and run an errand at the drop of a hat. I didn't mind being "driven." It was nothing like giving up dancing!
I liked our van even though we both had set our sights on a different kind of vehicle. Instead of buying the Lincoln deluxe sedan Wayne had wanted for years, he graciously settled for a van that could be fixed up with a hydraulic lift,

and was the kind of conveyance that would accommodate my Classy Chassis after the removal of the passenger seat.

> *July 11, 1990*
>
> *Larry flew in from Wisconsin where he is an associate professor at the university, to help us make an assessment of our situation and give thought to future needs. He seems to put our lives back on an even keel.*

We had such a good time with our son and after he left, we felt the usual letdown. It seems that we delight in the distractions that come into our lives in order to get away from ourselves. For just a brief moment I allowed myself to wallow in self pity, wondering why I should even get out of bed. Then the phone rang and changed everything.

Through the Portland Muscular Dystrophy Association, KMTV Channel 12 asked Wayne and me to take part in the upcoming Labor Day Telethon. I had been watching the Jerry Lewis telethon with special interest for years because each event raised large amounts for research on forty types of muscular diseases, one of which is ALS. Here was my chance to participate, perhaps even make a difference in somebody's life.

To my question of what was involved in appearing on the show, the director explained his crew would set up their equipment in our home and that the taping would take several hours.

I agreed readily. Each experience that comes your way is an adventure.

July 18, 1990
The big event!

Right on time, at one o'clock in the afternoon the door bell rang. Wayne opened the door and greeted the director with his crew of four technicians, each carrying an armload of equipment, all looking very hi-tech to me.

With professional savvy, the crew descended on our living room with the air of a well trained army assault unit — moving furniture, checking lights and angles, and before we knew it, the room was transformed into a television studio. Miles of cable crawled along the floor; a huge umbrella light bore down on us, bright lights were placed at every angle. All the while Sara, the pleasant young blonde interviewer, sat on a high stool doing a warm-up; her soothing voice coaxed us to relax while lights were being rearranged, the audio tested and the photographer scurried about adjusting camera angles.

The taping began in our living room with Sara conducting the interview by asking pertinent questions yet maintaining a comfortable tone. My answers were generally preceded by an unnecessary, drawn out "Uh" while staring at the floor (my thinking pose) or sneezing violently — all of which had mercifully been edited out for the final tape. For a change of scene, we went into the kitchen where the camera zoomed in on Wayne putting a casserole in the oven. (He really does cook but his specialty is hamburgers, pork chops, or bacon and eggs.)

Leaning on my walker, I shuffled to my computer room where a crew member aimed his camera over my shoulder to record for all the world to see my expert thumb-and-knuckle typing method. It may have been degrading for a former crack typist to be caught typing with her knuckles, but it demonstrated how I was able to bring my thoughts to paper.

The crew recorded us strolling down the wooden ramp, the nose of my "Classy Chassis" bursting through the creaky wrought iron gate (we really should have had it oiled). The camera followed us on our short walk down the block, while the chief of "cutting and pasting" encouraged my chatter by listening to my rendition of tips for living — about making every moment count, doing the things I enjoy, threatening to leave my footprints on the path of my journey on earth.

Soon, the crew recaptured their black snake-like cables, folded the umbrella lamp, placed their cameras in leather cases and politely bowed themselves out the door. The equipment was loaded in their impressive-looking white van, emblazoned with big red letters, telling the world who they were: CHANNEL 12 - KMTV.

The following day the crew returned briefly to tape additional footage, including a scene where a friend used my cardholder to help me play my hand during a simulated bridge game. By then, I was a pro at that sort of thing, acting cool and nonchalant while my friends were quite in awe at being able to observe the inside workings of creating a segment of a television show.

I had a great time throughout the tapings, and was looking forward to seeing the results on my television set in September. But first, we would have to get ready for our Alaska adventure, which wasn't far off. We had invited our 22-year old granddaughter, Kristine to join us, which, as it turned out, would be the highlight of the cruise.

Attractive, friendly and very pretty, she managed to get the attention of the ship's crew with her smiling face at every turn. We had superb service and Kristine was the center of attention, while I sat on the sidelines with Wayne enjoying every moment of it. The rest of the cruise was not as smooth as I had envisioned it. Let's face it, even my sophisticated, motorized do-it-all-go-everywhere Classy Chassis was not the kind of conveyance ideal for traveling the decks and corridors of a cruise ship on high seas.

As much as I loved our first cruise, I was glad to be home again this time. There are certain things we all give up for one reason or another in our lifetime, and there are a million things I could do other than cruising the oceans.

September, 1990
The Labor Day Jerry Lewis Telethon........hard to describe the emotion of watching one's self on TV. It's like observing a stranger and suddenly you realize, "That's me."

Wayne, Judy and Susan drove me to Portland where we watched the tapes for the Jerry Lewis telethon on TV at the local Muscular Dystrophy Headquarters in the Marriott Hotel. We settled ourselves in front of the monitor, anticipating a good show. However, in less than a minute into the tape of my story of living with amyotrophic lateral sclerosis our emotions were getting raw.

Eight-year old Susan held my hand and said, "I'm lucky to have a grandma like you." That did it. Tears spilled over, and I realized I was the fortunate one — regardless of circumstances — to have a wonderful, loving family.

Several months later at an awards dinner given by the Muscular Dystrophy Association we were surprised with another viewing of the tape. An "Inspiration" plaque was presented to me. "What some people won't go through just to get a plaque," was a snide remark heard at the far side of our table. I knew that the remark was made in jest — out of heartfelt empathy and emotions too strong for straight talk.

The most important aspect of this entire episode was that more people heard about ALS. Although the disease has been around for 100 years, little is known about it, and it may take another 100 years to find a cure. It had remained obscure until baseball great, Lou Gehrig made his impassioned speech in the 1930s. That was 60 years or so ago. The bulk of the research for finding the cause and cure has only been done in recent years.

In 1993 it was believed that a defective gene was the cause of the disease. In familial ALS the disorder is associated with chromosome 21, according to information released by the Muscular Dystrophy Association. That discovery was a start and probably the most important find to date.

ALS is a relatively rare disease, with statistics vacillating between one person to four in 100,000 having the disease at any given time. The variation is due to the fact that the life span of an ALS victim after diagnosis is usually short. The disease is caused by certain nerves emanating from the spinal cord failing to activate muscles. The gradual degeneration of muscles leaves the victim completely helpless and ultimately paralyzes the swallowing and breathing muscles until death provides relief.

Once the thoracic area is attacked and immobilized, there's little left that resembles life. So far, I have been incredibly fortunate that the weakening and destroyed muscles are restricted to my arms and legs.

September 8. 1990
I had a real jolt yesterday when I could not rise from the chair which I use at my computer. A sign of

things to come? In the meantime, I must keep on typing. I have work to do.

I've had practice, I have learned that there is an answer to every question, a solution to every problem. When one thing fails, several new ideas are waiting in the shadows to be given a try. The patent office of the United States Government is spilling over with people's inventions clamoring for patent rights. There are no "patents" given for inventing new and different ways to cope with life's little surprises — you just do it, and the world is yours!

I called my good friend, Mary Alice, whose innovative ways always amazed me. She studied the room where I did my writing for a moment, and started to move furniture around, until she was satisfied she had arranged things so that I could get to my work station in my "space-claiming" Classy Chassis, remaining seated in front of the computer with the keyboard firmly settled on my lap. This arrangement would work until I had to face whatever happened next.

It's a challenge to stay ahead of the game.

November, 1990

Back to back house guests: Ana and Jorge from Costa Rica, then niece Marilyn and Ed. Visitors had always been part of life — a wonderful part before ALS — and we shall continue to enjoy guests as long as possible. All it requires now is more help in the house. Our favorite holiday, Thanksgiving is around the corner and I am having difficulty getting up off the bed. My unpredictable legs are forsaking me.

December 20, 1990
We had a 17-hour power outage. Another adventure? Hardly — just a nuisance.

Christmas week started off with a bang. It was eight o'clock in the evening when Wayne and I had settled comfortably in our cozy living room enjoying our favorite TV show. Suddenly — total darkness. We waited. "It will probably come back on in a few minutes," we assured each other optimistically. Actually, it took 17 hours before the lights came on again.

Wayne fumbled his way to the closet through the pitch-dark hall, found a flashlight and lit the gas log in the fireplace, both for warmth and the glow of light. The room was getting chilly and I decided to get up to move closer to the fire. I pushed the lift button of my electric chair. Nothing happened. I had forgotten that my (lift) chair was "wired" to an electric outlet and without electricity it was as movable as a rock set in cement. Here I was stuck in a supine position, my feet sprawled outward and upward — possibly confined for the night. Wayne called a kind neighbor, who hurried over at once. When he saw me in my awkward position trying to look unconcerned and nonchalant, he could not suppress a grin and soon we were all laughing at my predicament.

Together the two men pushed and tugged at me, and finally, with a mighty heave-ho got me on my feet and settled me onto my scooter in front of the fireplace, still chuckling.

I'll never be able to say enough about the healing magic of laughter. Being able to look at one's miseries, one's limitations — imposed, self inflicted or otherwise — equalizes, re-evaluates and refreshes heart and soul.

Another lesson, another tweak on the cheek — laughter IS the best medicine!

There was still no electricity at bedtime, and we piled covers on top of us — just like years ago on a wintry night on the farm. It was not until the next afternoon that power was restored, and we marveled at how we had become accustomed to all the comforts of modern life.

Christmas 1990
SNOW! Six inches of beautiful, fresh snow ... pristine and pure.

We rarely have measurable snow fall in our area, and consider it a super bonus if it snows at Christmas time. The view from our back windows resembled a New England picture postcard. The tall firs were covered with a white blanket, bowing their snow-laden branches as if in prayer. Our little world was serene and calm, still and quiet, and brought peace into my heart.

Family and friends gathering during the holidays gave us yet another wonderful season, and we enjoyed every breath of it. Wayne and I love it when our home is filled with people sharing in the festivities, and enjoying themselves, the food, the fun and each other. Sometimes I think we don't do enough celebrating. We get bogged down by daily irritations, annoyances and "busy work" and don't take enough time to honor the very essence of life, each other's gifts and talents. There is nothing more enriching, more healing than a room echoing laughter and merriment.

Laughter breaches the gap between sorrow and disappointments and holds together the fragile structure of daily living. The whole world needs to practice laughing a lot more.

New Years Day, 1991

I am worried ... concerned ... not happy. Must resolve to be in a better frame of mind. The realization that I can do less and less makes me fretful and concerned about the future. My general mood was nothing to brag about. I must follow my own advice — and laugh.

Jan. 8, 1991

Larry flew in for a six-day visit and brightened our world with his cheerful presence and constant support.

He took me shopping, we drove here and there, and did a lot of other fun things. Wayne, Larry and I discussed our future and speculated what it might hold in store for us. In spite of all the deep thought, speculations and tentative planning, trying to foresee all the "what-ifs and what-thens," was about as effective as reading tea leaves — and just about as accurate.

I kept reminding myself that if everything we ever worried about would have come true — why, we wouldn't be here at all!

Larry read my half-finished manuscript, *Voices of the Prairie,* and encouraged me to keep on writing, even though I sometimes wondered who in the world would want to read it. Father and son checked out my equipment and ordered a new (five-inch) taller toilet seat than the one we had. Getting up and down from any sitting position was something I had never thought of as a special human feat — until ...

I thought about what I had taken for granted, all the inconsequential "little" things I no longer could do for myself, and as I started ticking them off mentally, I stopped as quickly as I had started. There was no profit in doing that. What would it accomplish?

So what if my fingers couldn't work with clay any longer — I never did anyway. Nor did I crochet, knit, sculpt, paint in oils, refinish furniture, build houses, repair bicycles, sky dive, lay pipe, hang paper, repair watches or hoist sails. And that list was just a beginning!

I realized that I had given up less than I ever did anyway, and I've called this act of mental acrobatics my "Blue Smoke Exercise" and got so good at it, that I could teach it.

In my reading I came across something which gave me a lot of comfort and food for thought. Julia Seton wrote:

"Life has taught me that it knows better plans than we can imagine, so that I try to submerge my own desires, apt to be too insistent, into a calm willingness to accept what comes, and to make the most of it, then wait again. I have discovered that there is a pattern, larger and more beautiful than our short vision can weave."

So be it.

February 16, 1991

I notice that my energy runs out quickly. I cannot spend much time working on my computer and am unable to do more than one social activity per day. It really isn't all that bad, is it now? I have had ALS for seven years and am grateful to be able to continue a relatively "normal" life. As the disease progresses, I am certain I will look back and realize what seemed so devastating at the time, really wasn't that bad.

One gray and soggy day a bright ray of sun appeared on the scene when Nella brought two dozen Thank-You letters written by the fourth graders of a grade school nearby. I had been invited to talk about my book *Memories into Memoirs*. When I appeared in the classroom, all eyes were glued to my three-wheeler. I realized I would have to explain the reason I was on wheels, or they would not listen to a word about my book.

I went into a short discourse on ALS, its effects on the body and how my Classy Chassis enables me to "walk."

Their curiosity satisfied, I read story after story from my book to my young audience. They were fascinated to hear about growing up on a farm in such different times. They were surprised to hear that I had read and studied by the light of a dim kerosene lamp when I was their age, and walked a mile in knee-deep snow to get to school — it was all so foreign to children who grew up in a car seat in a push-button world.

When I left their circle of happy faces, I had the feeling that the children had given me more than I had brought with me. And, maybe I had planted a seed in their fertile minds about the pleasure of writing stories. The kids seemed all fired up about it — if only temporarily.

Sometimes when I feel I am not doing anything worthwhile, something comes along that proves me wrong. I was grateful for that day.

Rich experiences such as my visit with a roomful of eight-year olds, double in value in later life — especially when I am threatened with complete immobility in the future. I must grasp every opportunity to help others and thereby help myself.

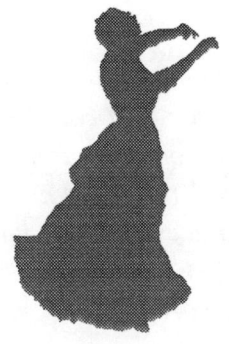

Chapter Eleven

*I keep plugging along and don't expect
to move mountains.
All I can do is to change
the perspective from which I view them.*

April 7, 1991
As I write this, I am totally frustrated. It has been raining for ten days and I'm in the house all day. My legs are weaker and I'm crabby.

When all else fails, I plan a party. I got busy and prepared a birthday party for one of our friends, who was turning 88. He was so very pleased and surprised. This simple act made me happy, made him happy and the 14 guests helping with the celebration were delighted.

Number One Lesson:
Get away from yourself.
Stop the gloom machine.
Do something for someone else. It pays dividends!

June 6, 1991
I am devastated! When I got up during the night, my left leg felt like it would crumble. It could very well be the end of walking. I fell apart. What to do? During the next couple of days, I rested frequently. It didn't help. My condition makes our life hard, with the certainty that it will get worse. Wayne is coping well, but the day-to-day care of me is wearing on him. We try to adjust our days to make sure he has a life of his own. His therapy is golf and he plays three or four times a week.

Before the howling howlies get the best of me, I switch gears — again. I "go" for a walk in my Classy Chassy by myself or with a friend. In bad weather I read a good book and get lost in someone else's trials and tribulations, as well as the joy and fulfillment the author's characters experience. I visit a friend, or someone comes to see me, and, I write. Writing silences my worrisome mind chatter, it is my refuge, my peace-bringing solace.

July 2, 1991
Larry and Lori came for a visit. Not only do they boost our moral, but they installed my new bed that raises my head and my feet at the push of a button. More aids for more ease. I am fortunate these gadgets are available.

When it was first suggested to me to install a motorized, adjustable bed, I was quietly horrified. In my mind's eye, I stomped my blue fuzzy-slippered foot and announced to myself: "I will not have anything that looks like a hospital bed in my bedroom. Just one look at a hospital bed makes me feel like an invalid, and I won't have that."

Fortunately, the most practical "hospital bed" came in a beautiful cherry wood, complete with a dust ruffle which concealed all of the iron workings underneath the belly of the bed, and had no resemblance to hospital equipment.

Setting up the bed presented quite a challenge to Larry and Lori. The bed came unassembled and arrived the morning of the same day they were scheduled to catch a plane to return to Wisconsin.

With six pages of instructions in hand, the two handy people began to assemble pieces of metal and wood. It did not take them long to discover that an important part of the bed part was missing — nothing less than the frame. Larry called the place the bed came from, and in no uncertain terms let them know the problem. Half an hour later the frame was delivered to our door.

Racing against the clock, the two of them calmly and smoothly plowed through the pages of instructions: fit part A into part B, (see illustration #56) etc. Racing against time, the air was electric with intensity and furrowed brows. The entire bed was put together with neither a nut nor a bolt left over. Perfect. Larry and Lori grabbed their suitcases and rushed to the airport. Well done!

July 11, 1991

An occupational therapist from Muscular Dystrophy Association came to teach me a new way of rising from my shower chair. It didn't work. My legs crumpled under me. Slowly and unceremoniously, I met the floor. Fortunately, due to the foresight of my husband and children, a hydraulic lift had been delivered two days before, just in the nick of time.

I knew this would happen sooner or later. Using my walker to take only the four steps from my bed into the bathroom had become a major chore. My legs trembled and wobbled like rubber bands and I had a terrible fear of falling with each step I took.

I felt somewhat ambivalent about my new hydraulic lift. On one hand I was glad because I no longer would have to rely on my legs to carry me and eliminate my fear of crashing on my way in and out of the shower. On the other hand, all feelings of dignity went out the window as I was being hauled around with feet splayed out in front of me like a turkey about to be stuffed.

First the walker, then my three-wheeler, followed by the motorized bed and now The Lift, all represented the cold, hard fact — the brutal reality — that I had become more and more dependent upon others, as well as requiring the aide of hospital equipment to maneuver me from point A to point B.

Carried on a strong, but brief breeze of momentary self-pity the windmills of my mind turned and tumbled my thoughts around and around. Well — hadn't I spent years and years of my life seeing to the needs of others? Hadn't I hauled and lugged, cajoled and soothed, fetched and carried? Shouldn't it be my turn now?

Wrong. That sort of logic was not for me. I've always had a deep need to be independent, but I also had the need to move on, to do and to accomplish what I could. If it had to be with help from others — so be it. It was a dilemma to which I had to adjust, and consider myself lucky to be surrounded by caring and loving people who not only helped me carry my load, but with grace and patience carried their own with only minor grumblings.

Again, I counted my blessings.

August 4, 1991
I am having another gallstone attack! Am waiting for the new laperoscopy method of surgery to become available in our area.

For three years I have been adhering to a low-fat diet in the hope of fending off a gall bladder operation. I had done my research on the less invasive surgical procedure (laperoscopy) and hoped it would soon be available. I watched and waited, until now. The procedure was being done in Portland. Lucky for me.

August 12, 1991
Doctor Keith Holmes removed my gall bladder by the new laperoscopy method. How miraculous! It could be called band-aid surgery. Only four small incisions were required for the removal of a problem gall bladder. One of my friends said, "You make the odds come out even."

Only a week after surgery I was able to go shopping with Betty for four hours, in spite of everything. Even though I was completely worn out I enjoyed myself. Fatigue is at my side all the time, I just won't give in to it so readily and make the hours count.

I did make the best of each day, and time just flew — summer rushed into fall with the holidays on the heels of a bright and warm Indian Summer. I neglected my journal, gave my soul-searching and questioning, fretting moods a rest. I had no time for the blues.

November 1992
When I look down at my feet, I can't believe they're mine!

Sitting all day long in my chair, not being able to walk or exercise has severely affected my circulation. My feet and ankles are swollen beyond recognition. That's one of the side effects of immobility. Gradually my shoe size changed. No sooner would I get a few pair of new shoes that fit, my feet would outgrow them, and I would be looking for another set of shoes.

I was fortunate that my weight remained much the same. Apparently I could thank my metabolism for effectively burning calories in spite of the fact that I sat still all day and rested all night. I was just not moving around, and for several months now I had not been able to dress or undress myself. There went another slice of dignity and independence out the window.

At first I fought and grumbled and complained about being helped in and out of clothes. Nobody could do it right. Only I knew how to dress myself. That was all well and fine, except I was unable to pull on a pair of hose, fasten a bra, slip on a skirt or shrug myself into a shirt — never mind buttoning it.

Incredible. I couldn't believe it. Somebody had to dress me like a baby, turning me over, bending me here and there, tugging and pulling at my uncooperative body, whose suppleness resembled a sack of sugar. It took me a while to make an uneasy peace with the latest development, accept what came my way and be grateful that I had such kind and patient help who didn't listen to my grumbling, and with gentleness and compassion took care of my needs.

When it comes to being grateful — I say my thanks

everyday when I hear of people in their thirties and forties being diagnosed with ALS. I was lucky; I was almost 65 years old when the first symptoms of the disease appeared. Although I certainly didn't feel "old" — 65 is no longer middle age — it's more like being called mature. We have been told that "things go wrong" as we get older — so "they" say. Of course I hadn't expected for things to go that wrong.

New Year's Day, 1992
I just know it is going to be a fantastic year! Planning our 50th anniversary party ... checking into a new computer more suited to the lessening strength in my arm.

Finishing the manuscript for *Voices of the Prairie* was at the top of my priority list. After three years of research, coupled with my painstakingly slow way of getting my story on paper, riddled with self doubt (whatever made me think I could write a book?), it was time to banish my negative thoughts and get on with it. After all, how could I know if the book was any good or not, if I didn't write it? Encouragement from friends helped me to plug away.

I can only fail if I don't get started.

Another problem surfaced: It had become impossible for my hands and arms to operate the mouse of my computer. My friend Skip who knew a lot about computers, recommended the purchase of a new Macintosh Classic II with an extended keyboard which would serve my needs. We went ahead with the purchase, but I was a bit apprehensive about having to learn a new set of tricks to operate my new Mac.

February 17, 1992
I do get frustrated with my new computer, and when I am baffled to distraction, I call Skip, who helps me out of the jam. I think I'll put him up for sainthood — he would howl with delight at that preposterous thought. Besides, the canonization period is too long.

With lots of help and tons of patience from all parties, I soon learned to master my new Mac — so vital to completing my project. As I drew closer to the end of my story, my excitement grew.

Then came the epilogue.

Finis — except for revisions, of course.

I never dreamed that in spite of my condition, I would be able to complete a 30,000-word book by using a pencil, eraser-side down with my left hand supporting my right. Like a blind woman finding her way with her cane — tap-tap-tap — so had I tapped my way, a letter at a time.

The urge to accomplish my goal and staying steady on my course were the underlying forces that propelled me daily to my place in front of the computer, and disregarding discomforts and fatigue, moved that pencil from letter to letter, word to word, with unrelenting drive.

Next came the search for a publishing house that would accept my manuscript. I sent my "precious" writing to three literary establishments and waited with bated breath. I wasn't that naive as to think that a publisher would be clamoring for my first literary effort. But I had hoped that someone would be interested in *Voices of the Prairie*. After all, it was a true story, written in novel style, tracing my immigrant ancestors' perilous journey from Germany to the bare prairie of Nebraska Territory. Didn't that subject fit the profile of millions of Americans whose ancestors settled this land?

Were these publishers daft? They certainly didn't see it my way. Rejection slips for my manuscript arrived daily in spite of my objections. Not willing to spend my days fielding rejections, I put the project on hold. The main objective had been achieved: I had finished what I set out to do. I had written a book. One day, there would be a way to put it into print. I was certain.

In the meantime I got on with my life, enjoyed another spring, a few games of bridge, and made plans for the big event of the year — our 50th Anniversary, the Golden one.

May 1992

I am having a great time making preparations for our anniversary party on June 13th. Friends were wonderful to help, and I so appreciated their devotion to us and to our celebration. But there was always the utter frustration of not being able to do it myself. I'm into name calling now. The latest word is "wicked". ALS is a wicked disease.

June 13, 1992
WE MADE IT TO OUR 50TH.

An eight-foot-long banner sprawled across the wall of our party room at the club, attesting to the fact that Wayne and Angela Riggs had happily survived the first fifty years of married life.

Scarred and bruised as we may have been, unsure of the future, the fact that we were alive and that we were enjoying life so very much, was remarkable. The fearful dark and the murky grey, the sad and the ugly all fell away in the glow of this special celebration.

Having all eight members of our family together under one roof would have been celebration enough. The biggest thrill was to see my granddaughter Kristine in my wedding dress and looking like a replica of me at age 22 on my wedding day. Brad was handsome in his grandpa's navy uniform. The two young people were our perfect stand-ins. How could we be so lucky? It must be part of the Great Plan.

July 1992
Time to get back to the business of publishing my book.

Publisher rejection slips continued to arrive at my mailbox. I sought an evaluation of my manuscript from Ursula, a professional editor. Would it be of interest to the reading public? "Yes, with editing and rewriting," she replied after a reading.

With a go-for-it attitude and the blessings of my husband, I decided to self publish. Spending the rest of my life counting rejection slips was not what I had in mind. Besides it bruised my soul — not to mention my ego.

More determined than ever, I started on a new and unfamiliar path which led to one of the most exciting phases of my life. Ursula led me through the intricacies of publishing — from editing, to obtaining the ISBN code and the Library of Congress number, to designing the book and making arrangements for the printing, while rewriting, expanding and improving the manuscript.

During that time of doing what I loved, which

demanded my fullest attention, it seemed that I had put ALS on hold. I became more tolerant of the restrictions the disease had placed upon me. I was so busy, so excited, so passionately committed to my project, I paid little attention to myself — neither fretted nor worried, feared or despaired. I was too busy! Laughter may be the best medicine, but being busy runs a close second.

I also noticed that I had mercifully escaped colds, flu, sore throats and other nuisance health problems for some years. As a matter of fact, I had considered myself very healthy. I began to wonder if my positive attitude, my constant vigilance to drive out negative thoughts and emotions, and my refusal to give in and give up, had not favorably influenced my immune system. Was this possible?

Psychoneuroimmunology — the mind-body-connection — has been a most vital research project for years, and most of the research results point to the fact that the mind, indeed, is the control for the body's actions. Although I wouldn't venture a guess, I was fascinated with the possibilities, I read up on the subject, and continued to keep an open mind. I learned to never say never.

July 27, 1992
Meeting to approve final cover design.

How exciting to see an idea come to live, a dream come true and a goal reached. The cover for my book had been created by combining two old photos from the homestead farm with good graphics — it looked wonderful and eye catching.

Next came the tedious job of proofing and proofing and re-proofing to catch the things we missed on the first and second go around — again and again.

Done! Now I would have to wait several weeks before I could have a book in hand.

October 8, 1992
Today Voices of the Prairie went to press.

My editor suggested a print run of 1,600 copies. I almost fell off my cart. How could she toss out a preposterous figure like that when I was sure we could not sell two hundred? Maybe three hundred at the most. She, who may know a lot about publishing books and things, was obviously out of her head — 1,600 copies indeed!

I had written my story primarily for my family — a legacy, a gift, from the past for them and the generations to come. I never dreamed it was to touch the hearts of hundreds of readers throughout the United States whose forebears had immigrated to America under similar circumstances to those narrated in the book. It was a story based on facts to which a lot of people could relate.

Nov. 20, 1992
My books are here. What a thrill.

The doorbell rang. A young man stood in the doorway in a neat brown uniform and announced smartly: "I have some books for you." A simple enough statement — as if he were telling me the time of day. What followed was a deluge of 22 boxes of books being stacked at our front door.

It was overwhelming. I yo-yoed between ecstasy and panic. I was thrilled to have realized a dream, but I worried how we would ever sell all these books. We took pictures of this mountain of boxes stacked as high as the doorway, and looked around for places to store them.

We stashed them everywhere — in the corners of the bedrooms, in the living room, under a table, and we covered a few stacks with a beautiful cloth, and one of my treasured old hand-pieced quilts and called it nouveau art.

We had several hundred pre-publication orders to fill. Each book had to be autographed and mailed in time for Christmas. Wayne became a master at packaging and shipping. Before the month was out, we had disposed of three hundred and forty-five books, and within a year's time had sold all but one box of Voices of The Prairie. I considered our publishing venture a howling success.

Last day of 1992
This past year was one of the most exciting and gratifying one of my life. and the "villain" ALS , the wicked disease, has been the driving force behind turning my dream of publishing my book into reality.

Writing, publishing and selling a book was one thing, but there was a bonus that went with the project I never even dreamt about — the response to this simple little book was overwhelming. Letters poured in from all over the country from people I never met or knew. Some of the letter writers had their roots in Nebraska and their ancestors also had been pioneers on the land. Others had grown up in other parts of the country in similar circumstances, and we shared the same background.

Local newspapers interviewed me, articles popped up in major Nebraska papers, and the grocery store, Sack & Save in my hometown of West Point, Nebraska, sold carton after carton of books at the store's checkout stands. Local girl made good!

My friends gathered around, bought books and helped

celebrate, people arranged for autograph-signing parties, and showered me with their attention.

I felt I had a fan club out there — modest in numbers but high on praise. Readers were generous with their compliments and thank-yous, and took the time to write wonderful letters. I heard from old school mates and acquaintances I had not thought of in decades. Voices of the Prairie had bridged the years and brought us together again.

My family were my publicists and I purred with pleasure and bathed in the glow of the limelight. What can I say, I loved it all. My three-wheeler had changed into a chariot and I had won the race.

I was on a real high and I swear, the excitement, the activities, the response had turned into some magic chemistry in my body that seemed to halt the disease's vicious progression — at least for a while.

Someone once said: " Start with doing what is necessary; then what's possible. Soon you will be doing the impossible."

The hardest task is to eliminate the word "can't" from the thinking process, but once it is done, you can fly.

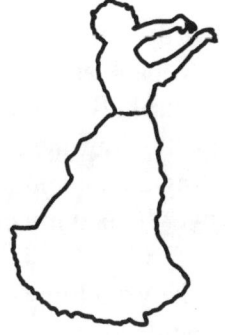

Chapter Twelve

*Life is so startling,
it leaves little time for anything else.*
Emily Dickenson

January 1, 1993
The new year brought us snow. If only the blanket of pristine whiteness could cover us and make our problems disappear, just as it turns the landscape into a different world.

But when it comes right down to the truth, I had to admit to myself that the blanket of snow didn't make anything go away — it only covered it up — everything is still there, just buried and hidden for a while.

Amyotrophic lateral sclerosis was still there under the blanket of my skin, eating away at my muscles, ready to pounce under the thin coverings of my home-made courage and serenity.

And, pounce it did.

I couldn't turn over in bed. I discovered that in a "normal" person the body moved voluntarily during sleep and repositioned itself from side to side, to back and front. But for the ALS patient, this common, natural body activity no longer works. Wayne reversed my position during the night which must have been equal to handling an unyielding sack of cement. An air pocket mattress cover helped my circulation and made turning easier.

All the moaning and groaning, the grumbling and the complaining did not help. All we could do was adjust to each situation and meet each challenge head-on, and keep going.

I liked to think I was living with ALS rather than dying with it.

It is the most wretched of diseases; it encroached on my muscles, gnawing away on healthy tissue like hungry termites on sturdy wood, until the muscles lose their strength and vitality, and the body is reduced to a shrunken mass of directionless flesh.

Eventually it robs the afflicted of the ability to swallow, eat and finally, breathe. It leaves the body unable to function until death provides the ultimate relief. Through all this degradation, the mind remains clear, alert and aware of the desperate circumstances, which place the care of the patient in the hands of others.

The advance and the effects of ALS differ for each victim. There is no set time, no schedule, no clock to watch on how the disease progresses — the prognosis is vague. Each person reacts differently and develops his or her own schedule of deteriorations.

Some people are afflicted with the bulbar type — paralyzing throat and breathing muscles. Others, like me, begin by losing strength in arms, hands and legs, caused by a growing deficiency in the nerves emanating from the spinal cord. In my case, it had been ten years since I was diagnosed. So far (thank heavens), I had been spared the encounter with the bulbar type of ALS.

January 14, 1993
Another January, another winter day, and it's snowing. Big, beautiful, downy flakes scatter on the wind and the temperature is down. If only cold feet were my biggest problem. I now have difficulty raising a cup to my mouth. I use a straw and bend my head to reach it. Difficult to eat a sandwich, even using both hands. What a bummer.

February, 1993
Letters! I get so many wonderful letters from readers who have enjoyed Voices of the Prairie. How flattering!

Each day's mail brought a new surprise - letters from cousins I had not seen nor heard from in forty years, visits from relatives near and far, all very precious to me. Someone wrote, "You have spent your time in a meaningful and lasting way. Your book will live on as a tribute." Words like these kept the delicate balance between self-esteem and worthlessness afloat.

Being dependent on your mate and on other people to be your designated arms, hands and legs easily deflated the spirit. The one and only way to get out of my periods of blue funk, was to get busy, and do what gave me pleasure, filled a yearning and had meaning. My passion is writing. I felt so fulfilled, so busy and occupied when I wrote *Voices of the Prairie*. It was an all-encompassing task.

Well, I could always write another book!

I gave it some thought, tossed the idea around in my mind and decided to write about living with ALS — what it is like to face a future which is bleak and despairing; I wanted to explain what it takes not to give in. I wanted to write a book that spoke not only to ALS victims, but to anyone who had been robbed of leading a "normal" life.

Just thinking about doing another book gave me a thrill, and the excitement and anticipation gave me a boost and made my spirit soar. By golly, here was my answer. I even came up with the working title of *Wrestling the Dragon*. Maybe it would later be changed, but for the time being, it would do.

> *March 4, 1993*
>
> *I notice that I can do less and less with my arms — the muscles are degenerating — slowly but surely. God, please help me to keep on being able to feed myself. As it is, I have food and drink clustered close to the edge of the table, like a mother hen with her chicks about her. Woe to the one who moves papers and tissues — even one inch will keep things out of my reach. That makes me think nasty thoughts ... but I hardly ever scream.*

I kept the fires burning under that driving force to accomplish as much as possible before my muscles turned into an inert mass of pulp. I still had the ability to make a difference — somehow. I willed myself to push on.

I was compelled to work on my manuscript, write a letter, or pour out my thoughts onto the patient pages of my journal. Anything, to leave my footprints behind, no matter how faint.

March 25, 1993
An hour before dawn (5:34 a.m.), my electrically-controlled bed started rattling like a tin can half full of marbles. It turned out to be an earthquake! — the first one for me.

Assuming the rattle was a power surge that made my electrically controlled bed go bonkers, I let out a piercing yell. Grandson John happened to be spending a few days with us and had just completed a study of quakes in eighth grade at school.

"Be calm. It's only an earthquake," he declared in a take-charge voice as he bounded out of bed and headed for the nearest doorway for protection. The only damage to our house in the earth's upheaval was a coffee server which fell off a shelf and landed a few feet from John's head. At the epicenter, fifteen miles away, the damage was a bit more extensive. Among the damaged buildings was a 100-year-old Gothic church in Mt. Angel, which ironically was the name of the fault.

Easter Sunday, April 11, 1993
Rain and lead-gray skies dim the bright colors of the spring flowers outside my window, just as they dim my spirit.
Strange how we react to the weather, how it influences our moods. I must guard against becoming "gray and murky." I can't change the weather, but I can change my outlook.

Change, change and more change. About the time I had become somewhat adjusted to the insidious surprises the current status of ALS had presented me with, another phase of muscle degeneration would make itself known posing new problems. Our warehouse of out-dated equipment was proof enough of the progress of the disease.

Through ten years of "experiencing" ALS, I had progressed from the use of one cane to two, to a walker to a three-wheel scooter. In addition to this variety of hardware we accumulated no longer serviceable shower chairs, a hydraulic lift and toilet seats — ranging from one inch in height to six inches.

Staying flexible and adjusting to changing demands with the least bit of grumbling was a must. A friendly face, a ready smile and a cheerful attitude helped my caregivers and my family to survive.

Whenever I put myself in Wayne's shoes, I saw clearly the enormity of his burden. I knew what his anticipations and plans for our "leisure" years had been, and I shuddered when I thought about the disappointments that had come his way. He may have grumbled a bit at times about some little annoyance, at some inconsequential bother, but when it came to the "biggies," he was at my side — he is great.

Marriages without strong foundations, without expressed respect and appreciation of each other's gifts, rarely survive crises and catastrophes. A good marriage overcomes everything. In our new world, of disposable goods and disposable people, we have lost the "stick-to-itiveness," the dedication to principles, the grace and strength of heart to rise to challenges. I am so blessed with my sturdy mate — my hero.

In spite of everything, I must say that we still had a very pleasant life, and part of that stemmed from the fact that neither Wayne nor I were bitter about our fate, quarreled with God and the world or took our disappointments out on each other as well as on others. People enjoyed our company, friends and family surrounded us with their love, surprised us with their thoughtfulness and never turned away from us. None of it was easy, it took work.

It is only human nature to fuss with fate, nobody wants to settle for less than what he expected life to be. Rarely do we appreciate what we already have, and we scheme and plan the future and expect our dreams to come true and fill the longing in our hungry hearts. But — there are no guarantees in life and we better learn to cherish the moment, because the future is just that — promises, hopes and dreams.

And then, all of a sudden disaster strikes. It seemed God had turned his back on us. The promises were false ones — there was no rainbow and God left by the back door.

I discovered soon into the game of life that there were no dividends in grumping up a day, and there was no profit dealing in gloom and doom. "Cry and you cry alone — Laugh and the whole world laughs with you." I had heard that one before!

A poor-me attitude wasn't worth the powder to blow it up. The longer I practiced cheerfulness, the harder I tried to make accommodations with my condition, the more I let the world see a smiling face and the more I watched the words that came out of my mouth, the better I got at it.

It may be blue smoke — BUT IT WORKED.

July, 1993
Losing strength in my arms daily. I love having lunch with my friends, but it's getting to be quite a problem just to bring the sandwich up to my mouth. I feel like such a klutz.
So why am I fussing about the mechanics of eating when I did lunch four times this week with

friends? God willing, I'll continue to be a player, not a victim who waits out the game on the bench.

I kept talking to myself long enough and was surprised how well I listened to my rhetoric. My arms and my hands rested almost lifeless and heavy in my lap, the battery in my legs had worn out, but the rest of me was healthy and alive. My head was full of ideas and there were still dreams in my heart. That was a lot more than some people had.

July 30, 1993
Wayne's 78th birthday. Cause to celebrate his good health.

We did celebrate the day with friends and family and had a grand time. In spite of all the major health problems he went through, living with some of the not-so-pleasant after effects of surgeries, the silver hair and the lines of living criss-crossing his face, he stood as tall and straight as the young man in his navy uniform of more than 50 years past and was just as handsome. It was indeed a happy birthday.

I had not been able to walk for two years. It was time for me to become accustomed to the routine that took me from point A to point B — the nylon sling being hooked up to the chains of the hydraulic lift to carry me from chair to my three-wheeler — or anywhere else for that matter. I felt like a rag doll. I seemed to be tense constantly, which did not help my husband one bit. If I could go for a 25-minute walk the knots in my stomach would go away.

Strike that! I would have to feel better without going for a walk with my legs. A spin in my three-wheeler wasn't so bad after all, I kept reassuring myself, and a piece of my favorite candy would hit the spot.

August 9, 1993

I have a better outlook on life again since Larry and Lori came for a five-day visit and moved mountains. Whenever life becomes too chaotic, new patterns emerge — so I've learned the hard way.

Those two young people came into our home like a fresh ocean breeze, looked at my situation and got the picture quickly. They immediately spotted the source for my depletion of strength, which they suggested (correctly) might be conserved with the help of a newer, more sophisticated conveyance that offered a stronger back support than my present scooter.

Was I ready to give up my faithful Classy Chassis? The one decorated by my artist friend, featuring hand-painted flowers and a sea gull that soared high, just as my spirit was supposed to? The thought was inconceivable.

"A power wheelchair would save your strength for the things you like to do," they both reasoned.

There was that awful, offensive word again — Wheelchair.

No matter how stubborn I could be, I listened to my own voice inside me which told me they were right, and I gave in to reason.

Off to the medical equipment store we all went to go chair shopping. I was determined not to like any of them, and did not hide my reluctance until the top-designed-in-Sweden model was paraded in front of me. That whizz-bang, hi-tech chariot did about everything but fly — it stopped short, turned on a dime, backed up smoothly, and zoomed off again. WOW! This clever, mini-auto opened up a new chapter for me — one that predicted a pleasant ending.

We took the demonstration model home to try for a day or so to see how I would "take" to it.

The next 24 hours gave new meaning to the word Wheelchair which I had refused to utter for ten years. Technology had indeed marched on: I could sit in relative comfort most of the day in the new carriage. Four electric adjustments made it possible to change the portion of the chair that supported my midriff muscles, which were not much sturdier than a bowl of Jello.

Naturally, we ordered the chair, and it was delivered a few weeks later. This wonderful cart made an enormous difference in my life and in my outlook. I felt less restricted, more mobile and able to maneuver in places and corners that had been difficult to navigate before. But the machine was so extra sensitive to the slightest touch that it could be compared to a high-strung, skittish horse — one false move and I had a runaway on my hands. After bashing into furniture and, worse, bruising my feet, I confirmed what I already knew. I was not born to race.

In answer to my call for help, our friend Eric, who sold these machines, came to the rescue. He slowed down the controls of the vehicle and made it more suitable for a wimpy driver like me. He gave me a lesson on getting up the ramp to our van and boosted my self confidence in general. My new power chair lightened my life and gave me more freedom. IT and I got along well — we were a slick act.

Looking back at the procession of mechanical aids that have come and gone in the last ten years, I realize that we couldn't have done it without the help of the Muscular Dystrophy Association. Their services not only made us aware of the availability of equipment but more than that helped carry the financial burden. Being ill or "physically challenged" is not only a tragedy but a tremendous financial burden.

Wayne and I are both grateful.

August 27, 1993
Today I'm 74 years old and I am having the most fantastic birthday ever. When Wayne's Irish golf partner stopped by and learned it was a special day, he stood in the kitchen doorway and in his rich tenor voice presented me with his rendition of "Irish Lullaby."

Good friends brought cake and champagne, which resulted in a spur-of-the-moment celebration of life. The house rang with laughter and I felt like my old self again. Big bouquets of beautiful flowers and an armload of cards overflowing with good wishes made me feel blessed and cherished.

There were so many people who went out of their way to bring brightness and light into other people's lives — often at great cost and sacrifice to themselves. In these past years of difficulties and often devastating events, I was showered with affection and attention by people who just wanted to make me feel good and loved and cared for. Have they ever succeeded! I hope I am that thoughtful.

October 3, 1993
The hundreds of everyday, common little things we take for granted until we can no longer do them. The numbness and muscle cramping caused by being rooted in one and the same spot awakens me

from a sound sleep. Inching over to my back brings relief until Wayne comes in to roll me over. He has to do that two times a night. Adjusting the bed to have my head up, and feet down is a necessity. If only my arms will remain strong enough to operate the buttons.

It had been a while since we attended an ALS group support meeting. It wasn't for any particular reason that we skipped them for several months. Perhaps we wanted to ignore the real world for a while and remain within the more comfortable boundaries of our own making. I thought about the many people who belonged to one support system or another — from AA groups, to grieving, death, cancer and other types. We all wanted to reassure ourselves that we were not alone with our pain, but at the same time — off and on — we needed to stay away from groups for a while because of the constant reminder of our "problem" the group represented.

There were several ALS patients at the meetings who were in the final stages of the disease. Their faces portrayed a mixture of quiet despair, hopelessness and mute acceptance. One man always had a merry twinkle in his eyes, as if he had just heard a good joke and was trying to suppress his laughter. Overall, good humor, hearty chuckles and spontaneous laughter were no strangers in the room. We were all in the same boat — trying our best to keep it from turning over and drowning us in the dark waters of our despair.

No matter how we looked at our world, no matter how we resolved to banish our fears and make the best of life — it didn't come easy. It was work. But, it was good work. And the results brought peace and quiet pleasure into our hearts.

Wayne escaped to the golf course as often as he could manage, and I was always so glad to see him charge off. He carried a big load and found his release in the company of his buddies.

I would head for my computer, clasp my "typing tool" and get lost in my own world. No matter what stage of life in which we find ourselves, it so important to have something, some hobby, some activity in our lives that take us away from it all. You can let each moment be a reminder of your dilemma, or you can turn your back on it and do something constructive.

Oct. 12, 1993

A physical therapist from the Muscular Dystrophy Association came to demonstrate a method for getting in and out of bed and being hitched up to the hydraulic lift. My back is no longer strong enough to keep me upright so I can sit on the edge of the bed. It was a gruesome hour. I was being shoved, pushed, manipulated until I was physically and mentally exhausted.

Losing complete control of my muscles and forcing me to entrust the handling of my body to another person was fearful, as well as mentally devastating. There I was, a grown woman, being bounced about like a rubber ball, all the while chastising myself for being afraid.

"Afraid of what?" the voices inside me seemed to sneer — much as one would talk to a recalcitrant three-year old. "Well ..." My voice trailed off, too weak and ashamed to say that I was frightened about the idea of falling off the bed, an event which could not possibly happen with three grown people hovering over me. I should have taken a hefty tranquilizer before the therapist started her ministrations but how was I to know I was going to freeze up?

I never did get over the fear of being manipulated — not entirely.

Nov. 16, 1993
I'll mark this date in Red on my calender! Another experiment has been announced to determine the cause of ALS. I wonder...? I wonder? I wonder...?

In ten years of living with ALS, I have outlasted several clinical trials, which have come to naught, and have overused the word hope. Along with the other victims of ALS, I was grateful that research was still going on. The effort to make the public more and more aware of the disease continues in the hope that visibility and information will lead to raising the funds to keep on searching and experimenting until the answers are found. The secrets of many dreaded diseases have been unraveled, cures were discovered, and, in some cases, science has wiped a slew of cursed conditions off of the map of human suffering.

Four month, ago Dr. Patric Clapshaw of Kirkland, Washington took blood samples from ALS patients (our people from our ALS support group formed the nucleus for this experiment) as well as from corresponding non-patients. Test results showed a similarity in the blood make-up of those who were victims of the disorder.

The search continues and the word hope can still be found in pages of the dictionary.

Someday ... sometime ... it will come.

December, 1993
Time just flies, here it is winter and the Christmas month is upon us.

During that time of year, my thoughts are happy and memories bring back childhood Christmases on the farm in Nebraska. December weather was always cold and icy. A bitter wind whistled sharply across the wintry landscape blowing the deep snow into hills and valleys of white down. On those frosty, crisp Christmas Eves the nine of us piled into our 1923 Chevrolet, and Pa slowly and carefully maneuvered the auto over the snow-covered icy roads to the country church.

Our formal celebration of the season began with attending midnight Mass. The smell of incense and candle wax mingled with the pungent fragrance of pine boughs, and the hushed singing of Silent Night filled the little church and made for a peaceful feeling that everything was right in my six-year-old world.

I would be filled with a trembling excitement because I was certain St. Nicholas would bring me a present. Even if there weren't any "real" presents, an orange was sure to be on on my plate at the table, along with colorful hard candies and some pennies, a nickel or even a dime.

Sure enough, on Christmas morning, there it was — a big orange on each of our plates. The memory of eating the juicy fruit did not linger with me as much as the colorful picture of seven bright oranges glowing on seven plates — one for each child. Today, a common piece of fruit, these then exotic oranges were our once-a-year treat.

In the parlor stood a Christmas tree which our parents had managed to obtain from some corner of the treeless plains. The little tree was decorated with store-bought tinsel and red candles in tin holders were clipped to its branches. In the eyes of a child, it was sheer magic — it was the most beautiful tree in the world. Those were the carefree days of childhood, when I knew someone would always take care of my needs.

Life was simple then and expectations modest. (I wonder how our grandchildren would react to receiving an orange, a handful of candy and a few shiny coins in lieu of the fulfillment of their itemized list of toys, trinkets, Guess jeans and hi-tech gadgets?)

Times change and we can't stay in the past. However, it wouldn't hurt to revive and reinstitute some of the old and solid principles and attitudes from the past which served us so well.

Hello, 1994

I am thrilled that I have written 58 pages of my current book — "When The Music Stopped." When typing became too tiring I tried dictating into a tape recorder, but it didn't work for me. I guess I'm better at putting thoughts on paper than talking them to death. I feel more relaxed tapping away at my computer. I simply allow more time for the effort.

I really had hoped I could talk into a tape recorder to ease off on the time spent at the computer, but I found it was an additional emotional load. Writing it all down, going over what I had written was difficult enough as I retraced the events, thoughts, feelings, emotions and the unrelenting attack on my body as ALS destroyed healthy muscle tissue.

February 1, 1994

I am disturbed enough by my difficulty in getting

food to my mouth to have an occupational therapist visit, bringing utensils that might help with the feeding process.

Thanks to the resources of the ever on-the-spot Muscular Dystrophy Association, help is no more than a phone call away most of the time.

I now have a plate guard which keeps the food from going off the edge as I chase it around with my fork, like a dog hunting a rabbit in slow motion. My right arm gets tired before the meal is half over and I have to rest in between bites. I am unable to lift a cup to my mouth and drink through a straw. However, a cup of coffee loses some of its flavor when inhaled through that slim bit of plastic.

March 1, 1994
My joy in watching another Oregon spring unfold with the brightness and bang of a high-kicking chorus line was cut short by an emergency. Problems! A recurrence of Wayne's bleeding problem.

Just when things were going along quite well — Wham — a crisis occurred. At eight o'clock at night, (better than midnight) a kind neighbor had to drive Wayne to the hospital, where he was immediately given nine units of blood. Two days later he experienced angina pains. His doctors decided a double bypass was necessary. What a nightmare! Would he withstand one of the most invasive and taxing surgical procedures? My heart dropped to the bottom of my feet and stayed there while my prayers rose to the heavens.

Good News! Wayne made it. His strong constitution

carried him through.

It is hard to describe how we all worried and fretted and prayed and reassured ourselves. We could never have gotten through this crisis without the help of faithful Toni and Nella, my helpers, who did double time and dialed their fingers to the quick to find other helpers and friends who pitched in with the household chores as well as the caregiving. Our grandson John took over on weekends. Wayne was sorely missed while he recovered.

Wayne bounced back like a rubber ball, and in no time was his old self again. When I showed signs of depression during the aftermath, Larry helped me to get back on an even keel by reminding me to celebrate Wayne's happy ending and not resurrect the scary what-could-have-been phantoms. How true!

If I just kept on practicing what I preached to myself, I would catch on and would "walk" my talk. I would become my words and validate their meaning by my actions. Only then, could I expect others to follow my lead. Someone once said that words were lame and go on crutches, but actions had wings. I did want to fly.

I'd said it before and I'd say it again: The real hero in my life was Wayne. Caregiving is an art (and he was superb), one he learned by trial and error. If one approach didn't work we tried another — peppered with words not contained in Webster's Dictionary.

The main ingredient in caregiving is an inordinate amount of patience. My bedtime routine alone could try a saint to the limits of endurance. After helping me through a day of fetch and carry, of taking turns with Toni to tend to my personal needs (which include getting me out of bed and into the bathroom, showered, dressed and groomed), of picking up what I've dropped, bringing things into my reach that have escaped me, Wayne would nap peacefully in his favorite chair, relaxed like an old shoe. But not for long. Time to go to bed!

My evening program was the same as for anyone in the process of retiring for the night: Undress, bathroom, brushing teeth, grooming, and putting on sleeping attire. Most everyone could accomplish these things in his sleep — almost. Not in my case. It took me more than 20 minutes to complete the nightly chore.

With arms and legs as limp as a ragdoll's, undressing and dressing became a major tug-of-war. Then, when I was ready to be deposited on the sheets, Wayne hoisted me into the necessary position on the hydraulic lift — from here to there and into bed. My dear husband thoughtfully warmed up my bed with a heating pad to help revive my cold feet. My feet were always cold due to poor circulation and getting into a warm, cozy bed was the next best thing to heaven.

That wonderful feeling of being loved and cherished comes to full circle when Wayne tucked me in. There are no words for that. That moment always erases the negative thoughts about myself that come uninvited — when I don't like myself, when I quarrel with my fate and battle with my dragons, when I feel the burden of being a burden on the world, and finally, when I descend into the sinister darkness of my despair.

If only that terrible down-time would change my situation. But of course, it never does. It's just a waste of time when I could be doing something better. Someone wise once said, "If people would do to us what we do to ourselves, we would most probably kill them." It is not only kinder but it is easier to be a friend than an enemy, and I am learning to be my best friend and not my worst foe.

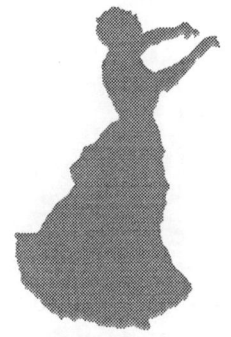

Chapter Thirteen

> I like living. I have sometimes been wildly,
> despairingly, acutely miserable, racked with sorrow,
> but through it all, I still know quite certainly
> that just to be alive is a grand thing.
> *Agatha Christie*

At the end of my ten-year run with ALS, I could count my blessings on one hand, while on the other I could not help but mourn the loss of physical functions and ordinary pleasures — simple things such as walking and, of course, dancing.

It is only human to grieve and feel sad at times. It's all right to cry and yell and shout in defiance over one's fate. But these moments of rebellion never lasted long and months went by without my falling into my woe-is-me mode. I could not deny my condition. I could not make-believe it wasn't so. It is, and I had to lump it and live with it. But the magic word was "L-i-v-e."

In spite of everything I could still love life and as long as I could live in dignity, I would stretch and reach and plan and do. I would cry and laugh, and rant and rave and celebrate that which is L-i-f-e.

But it has been the kind of life I chose to live. Life itself is fatal for everybody, and death is the last payment for the cost of having lived.

It is the end that differs, and the quality of the journey to reach that end.

I don't occupy my mind often with the idea of death, but I have given it some thought and have come to my decision. It may offend, disgust or horrify some people, but then they will be judging me from "where they are" — their healthy bodies and their personal views of morality

ALS is a horrid disease which slowly (sometimes quickly) causes the muscles in the body to deteriorate until they no longer function — like an overstretched, worn out, old rubber band, void of elasticity and strength. The victim is trapped in a shell of body, like a puppet whose strings have been cut, unable to move — raise an arm or a leg, lift the head, take a step. Even the most exclusively personal and private grooming chores — the things we do behind closed doors — are left to the care of others. No matter how I've tried to accept the help of others in these personal moments, I'm always embarrassed, mortified by the necessity of requiring assistance.

In so many cases of ALS, the thoracic area is one of the first sets of muscles to be affected and victims soon loose the ability to speak as the vocal chords become paralyzed. In the final stages of the disease, these unfortunate people can no longer swallow or breathe. Hooked up to a life support system which breathes for them in concert with a feeding tube to sustain what's left of their bodies, they are kept alive, imprisoned and mute in a tube of desensitized flesh. The only muscles still functioning in their once vital and mobile bodies are the ones which control the opening and closing of the eye lids.

Imagine the horror of being trapped like that, unable to utter a cry of protest, voice a plea to end the nightmare. Long before this final stage sets in, it is my strongest conviction that the family of the victim should have instruction from the afflicted persona as to what course to follow to end the misery.

This is what I want for myself.

I have no intention of inflicting an emotional burden on my family, to say nothing of the minute-by-minute care prolonged life in a soundless capsule would entail for them. That would be an enormous and unbearable load for everybody. I have no intention of being hooked up to a wheezing, gurgling, whirring set of machines to keep my helpless, inert body alive.

Alive — for what?

I love life too much to exist as a motionless hunk of blubber unable to do more than blink my eyes. The horror which I experience now as I think about ending up like this can't possibly match what would go on in my mind if I were put in such a terrible situation.

The simplicity of my upbringing, the respect for all living things and a deep appreciation for God's gifts are the foundation of my very being. Without patting myself on the back, I know that I have lived my days with dignity, and tried to be careful with people's feelings and alert to their needs. I have insisted on making choices for a productive, wholesome life, I want to have the right to choose the manner of my death. Some people may say that I will change my mind about that choice when push comes to shove. They predict that, true to human nature, I will cling to life regardless of the "lack of life" left in me. I don't think so.

I have arranged to donate my body to science in the

hope that it might aid researchers in their quest to find answers, prevention methods and/or a cure for ALS.

In November 1994, Oregon voters passed a law which enables physicians to legally assist in the death of terminally ill persons. In order to safeguard the integrity of the act, two physicians have to concur with the prognosis that the patient has six months or less to live. The request would have to be made by the patient — No One Else!

This unique law would make Oregon the first state to legalize physician-assisted dying — a way to end the suffering and indignities brought on by hideous, debilitating illnesses.

However, at this writing, the law has been put on hold and is being contested by those who feel that physicians should not have the right to assist in dying. All these contestants, no doubt, are healthy human beings whose idea of suffering is limited to an ingrown toe nail and the battle with a winter cold.

When the law finally comes to pass (again) it will give the long suffering the opportunity to choose between life and assisted death. They will be able to make the crucial choice: continue the agony or look for the relief that death can bring them. When the body is worn out — either by age or disease — we must be given the choice to release our spirit and be allowed to leave in peace, rather than live in hell on earth.

No one yet has lived forever, so why prolong living when all dignity is gone? I must also remember that I am no longer 60 or even 70 years old, and although I passionately protest my debilitating condition, I can imagine what it must be like to be struck down by ALS in the very prime of life. However, the suffering and the anguish, the loss of control and the hopelessness, the despair and the grieving are the same at any age.

Through our activities with our local ALS support group which is sponsored by the Muscular Dystrophy Association, Wayne and I have met ALS victims in various stages of the disease — none of them uplifting or pretty.

There was a man — about 50-years old — who was in the prime of his life and at the height of his career. ALS struck and took its toll quickly, soon paralyzing his breathing muscles. As with all victims, his mind remained clear, imprisoned in a helpless body. He and his family opted for the use of a respirator. After several months of endless misery, void of hope or relief, he made his last decision and asked for the respirator to be disconnected. Death brought the relief and peace life no longer offered him.

Another person stands out in my memory.

She was a pretty woman in her late forties. I approached her to inquire about her clothing which seemed to have been specially designed to adapt to the needs of wheelchair users. I discovered quickly that she was unable to speak. Her husband told me that the only part of her body she could move were her eyes.

Those beautiful, sad, brown eyes conveyed more feelings than words could tell. Their message came across like a bolt of lightning illuminating darkness. Her eyes spoke of kindness, compassion and an inner peace born of acceptance.

When I called her house two days later, I was told she had died and had indicated she wanted me to have her clothes. When the box arrived and I unpacked her lovely gifts, my eyes filled with tears, just as hers had only a few days earlier. Every time I wear her cozy, red wool cape which conforms so well to my body and fits the shape of my electric chariot, I see those soft brown eyes sending out their eloquent message of peace. That message will remain with me, always.

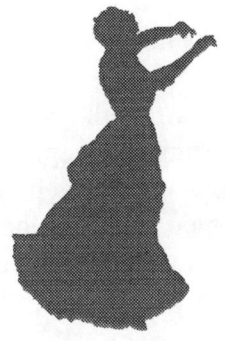

Chapter Fourteen

Difficult times are a reality —
but they come to pass.
Nothing comes to stay.

The saving grace in my life is my occupation with writing this book, even though I get discouraged about the increasing weakness in my right arm. Fatigue wraps me in a grey fog and cuts short my time at my computer. Sometimes, all I want to do is stretch out and close my eyes. However, I persist and I am determined to complete what I have started.

July 30, 1994
Today Wayne is 79 years old. He keeps reminding me of his advanced age, however I still think of him as my young athletic mate from 52 years ago.

Day after day, year after year, Wayne does so very much for me, and I must realize that he is entitled to become disgruntled now and then at the constancy of my dependence on him. I despise being caught in this trap of helplessness that we both bear and share.

Last night was an example of how thin the layer of his patience can wear. I had trouble getting to sleep. At midnight I decided I'd try a snack to put me to sleep. Wayne marched into the kitchen and returned with a handful of Graham crackers which he proceeded to feed me piece by piece, all the while shaking his head as if to say, "I can't believe I'm doing this."

As I've said the time it takes to get me ready for bed is especially trying and we both approach it with extreme caution. Usually, we are tired at the end of a day that most probably made heavy demands on both of us. We are on the edge of being cranky, and even an innocent remark can lead to disaster. It is best to keep the conversation to simple subjects like, "What time is it?" or, "It's cooling off a bit outside, I hope it won't rain tomorrow." Even that kind of general talk has the potential of causing dissension. It could. It is advisable for me to keep my mouth in a firmly closed position.

But when it's all said and done, Wayne deserves a Class-A blue ribbon on earth and a diamond-studded gold crown and wings in eternity. He's entitled!

August 27, 1994

Seventy-five and very much alive!

Birthdays seem to have more meaning as one grows older. I'm amazed that the accumulation of years has not changed some of the youthful feelings and notions I still have.

Yet, success achieved in later life is far more gratifying and meaningful than accomplishments in youth. Or is it the fact that not so much is expected of us in later years?

When I started this book one year ago it was on my list as a "possible." Presently, 137,000 characters later, these accumulating pages could be classed as a definite "probable." Considering my typing was done by dinking around with a pencil attached to the knuckle of my right hand and forced to rest after every few lines, the effort puts the hare and the turtle story to shame. But then the turtle goes forward only when he sticks his neck out.

Frustrations are the threads of which the cloth of my day is woven. They come and go and come back. The only variation is the degree of their intensity. They are born of simple things such as, "Give me a drink of water, please. I need a tissue, please. Hand me this book, thank you." I try to limit my demands in order to reduce the number of times I am forced to ask for help, making it less tiresome for Wayne and others.

It's amazing what I used to take for granted and what now fall in the realm of impossible:

Trying to retrieve a pen which has somehow jumped out of my hand. Grabbing for a book which mysteriously slid off my lap — with no muscle response to my mental command.

With great effort, attempting to turn to page two of the newspaper. (Actually, I don't get past page one.)

Looking for a letter somewhere under a pile of papers on my desk. Even if I could reach the letter, my fingers would not be able to grasp it.

Holding on to a slick magazine with the back of my hand didn't work too well.

The list is endless and gets bigger as the deterioration of my arm and hand muscles progresses. This was not intended as a laundry list of complaints, only an exploration of how minor actions which once were easy, now take on monstrous effort.

The words please and thank you are overused in my vocabulary to the point where my caregivers must surely be tired of them, but I would be remiss if I left them unsaid.

The hardest part is to let go of what used to be. Having to give up crafts, sewing, working, drying and pressing flowers — all that creative, busy work I liked so well and which required the use of finely tuned muscles of the hands. That of course was just part of it. I had to let go of a whole way of life, and that's all right. Resisting change, fighting petty battles and inconsequential issues, quarreling with life itself are all exercises in futility. I learned a long time ago that the only thing I can change is MYSELF. Once I understood that, I went to work on it, and practiced what I preached.

Have you ever wondered if patience improves with age? The answer is No. Instead I have learned to react to frustrations more wisely, gained a measure of peace and have found strength in the following words:

SYMPTOMS OF INNER PEACE

A tendency to think and act spontaneously rather than on fears based on past experiences.

An unmistakable ability to enjoy the moment.

A loss of interest in judging other people.

A loss of interest in judging self.

A loss of interest in interpreting the actions of others.

A loss of ability to worry.

Frequent, overwhelming episodes of appreciation.

Contented feelings of connectedness with others and

nature.
>Frequent attacks of smiling.
>An increased tendency to let things happen.
>An increased susceptibility to love extended by others as well as the uncontrollable urge to extend it.
Saskia Davis

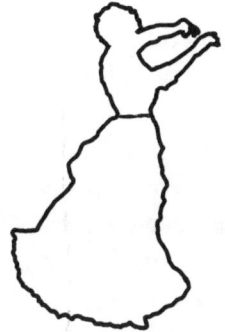

Epilogue

> Wherever your journey takes you,
> there are new gods waiting there
> with divine patience —
> and laughter.
> *Susan M. Watkins*

In these last eleven years, countless tides have washed over the wide shores of the Pacific Ocean and rushed out to sea again, leaving behind a scattering of driftwood, broken shells, silt, and seaweed. Underneath this rubble and buried beneath the smooth white sand hide the gifts from the sea — perfect, round sand dollars, multicolored stones polished smooth by centuries of turbulent waves, glistening pink shells that once housed living creatures.

Anyone who faces the bleak future of wrestling with a fatal disease must sort through the rubble in his life to find the elusive beauty that is always there somewhere — just waiting to be discovered. Treasure it. Cherish it.

Living with a debilitating condition has taught me many things, one of which is to expect the unexpected. With the degeneration of muscles on the rampage, there is a new development almost every day. Something may go wrong that had worked perfectly well the day before. One day I was able to put on my makeup, the next day I was teaching Wayne — of all people — and my caregivers how to fix my face...comb my hair...brush my teeth, put on my earrings, my necklace, my wrist watch or a bracelet.

The act of pulling on stockings, zipping up a skirt or buttoning a shirt went out the window right along with embroidering, darning socks or mending. There isn't room to list the simple things I can no longer do — and haven't been able to do for a long time now.

But the things I still can do would take up a lot of room: I can laugh and sneeze; I can breathe deeply of the fragrant blossom-scented spring air; I can smell the summer rain and the fresh breeze that brushes gently against my face; I can feast on the sounds and sights of Christmas; I can speak and even sing if I'd choose; I can read and write, go for a "walk" in my wheelchair, I can wrinkle my brow, shake my head, take part in conversations, cheer up and console others, I can, I can, I can ...

The real challenge in experiencing hardship of any kind, is to carry on and find a solution, a compromise and a mastery of the challenge. If the obstacle seems momentarily insurmountable at times, I call a friend, rent a movie, go for a ride, get a root beer float, buy myself some flowers, have a piece of candy, and above all, count my blessings.

I'm good to myself. I keep a box of See's chewy caramel-nut chocolates on hand in case of emergencies.

Be good to yourself!

I like taking part in the activities good friends invite me to share, I welcome fresh ideas from our grandchildren, although we are not always in agreement. I make demands on myself to keep my mind active and thrill to the simplest accomplishments rather than dwell on the frustrations and failures, which are always present.

The longer I live, the more I see. The more I see the more I learn. And, I have learned some invaluable lessons. I have learned that there comes a period in every life where people experience unprecedented hardship. Few people dance through life untouched by tragedy and heartaches. Without experiencing difficulties, life would be a steady diet of cotton candy. Compassion and understanding for others is born from personal pain and enriches our relationship with each other. And when the band stops playing, it is up to us to find a way to keep on dancing to the melodies that linger on in all of us.

For the third time now, I have begun my five-year life-death sentence that was handed down at the time of diagnosis. I have far outlived the statistics which attempt to describe the life span of ALS victims. The slow progression of the disease in my case is allotting me bonus time. Perhaps the game plan for my life ended in a tie, and therefore, I have been awarded extra innings. Whatever my purpose is, I intend to stay productive, treasure each day and, if I get rattled, have a piece of candy.

I have had time to reflect on the transition from this life to the hereafter. To me, heaven means seeing my mother and sisters again, being able to walk and walk and walk, and not ever having cold feet — ever. My octogenarian friend Neta Kaye looks upon dying as graduating to the next higher "grade" of being.

Believing in life after death is comforting. I think death is the equalizer to life and may well be a new beginning. As I have said before, our visit on earth is limited — some of us stay longer than others, and we live on in the hearts and minds of those we have inspired, and exist in our deeds. But by design of nature, the body finds a way to break down and stops functioning. There must be a million ways to leave this life, mine happens to be by way of ALS — at least that is the prognosis.

When that time comes, I will chose to follow the dictates of my mind and my body. Until then, I shall always hear the music of life with an open heart, listen to the lyrics of love with awe and wonder, and I will keep on dancing.

I'll keep on dancing.

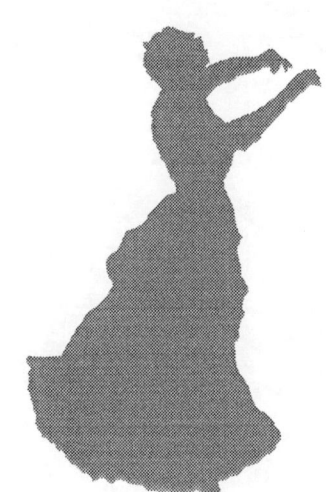

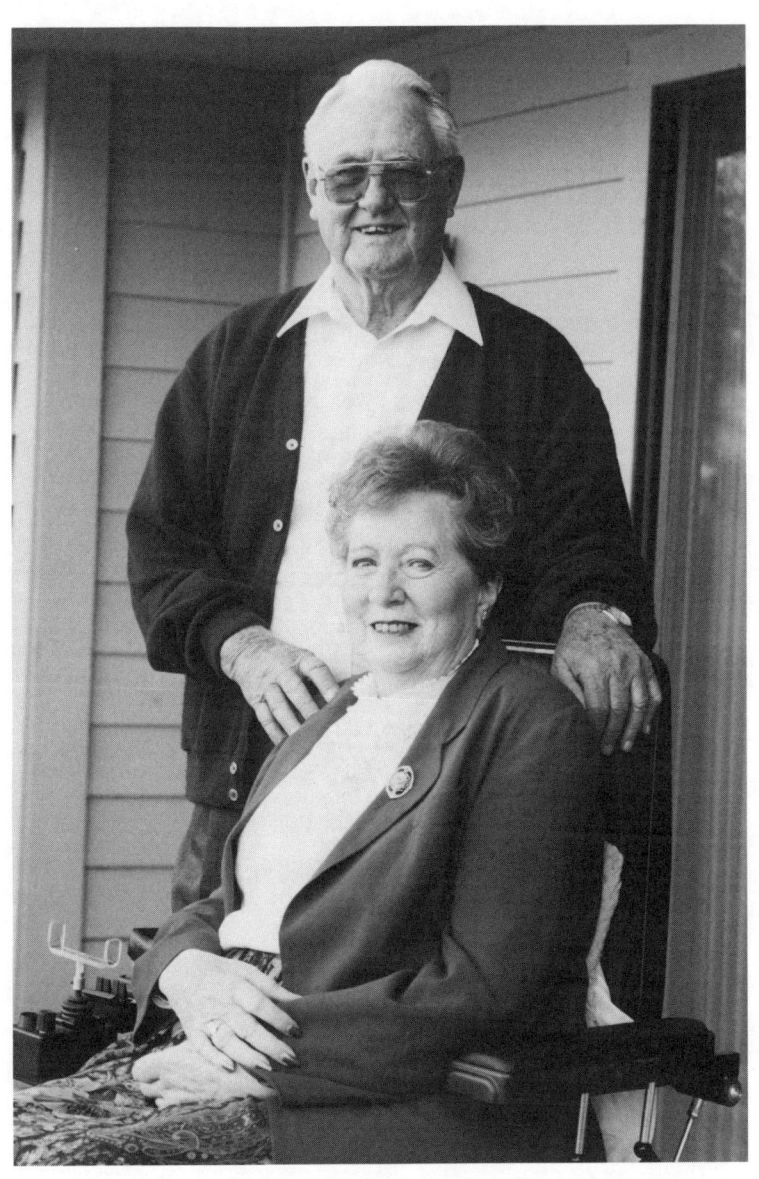

Angela and Wayne Riggs at home in Wilsonville, Oregon.

*Angela Riggs can be contacted personally
by writing to:*

*32465 S.W. Lake Point Court
Wilsonville, Oregon 97070*

To order additional copies of
When The Music Stopped
I Kept On Dancing

Please send ____ copies at $12.95 for each book, plus $3.50 shipping and handling for the first book, $2 for each additional book.

Voices of the Prairie. Please send ____ copies at $12 for each book, plus $3.50 shipping and handling for the first book, $2.00 for each additional book.

Enclosed is my check or money order of $_____
or [ ] Visa [ ] MasterCard
#_____ Exp. Date _____/_____
Signature _____
Phone _____

Name _____
Street Address _____
City _____
State _____ Zip _____

(Advise if recipient and mailing address are different from above.)

For credit card orders call:
1-800-895-7323

or

Return this order form to:

BookPartners
P.O. Box 922
Wilsonville, OR 97070

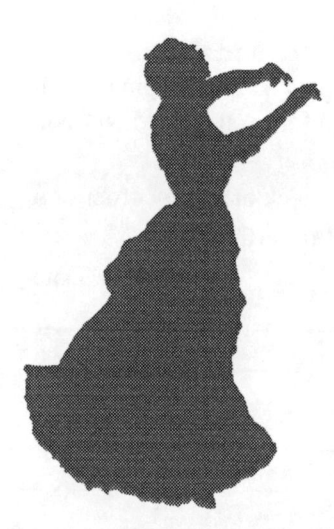